YOGA FOR MEN

REAL MEN DO DOWNWARD DOG

ind*i.e.* —
experts
IN OTHER WORDS

First produced 2021 by Indie Experts
PO Box 1638, Carindale
Queensland 4152 Australia
indieexperts.com.au

Cover design by Daniela Catucci @ Indie Experts
Edited by by Anne-Marie Tripp @ Dettori Publishing Pty Ltd
Internal design by Indie Experts
Typeset in 13/18 Adobe Garamond Pro by Post Pre-press Group, Brisbane

NATIONAL LIBRARY OF AUSTRALIA — A catalogue record for this book is available from the National Library of Australia

ISBN 978-0-6451019-0-4 (paperback)
ISBN 978-0-6451019-1-1 (epub)
ISBN 978-0-6451019-2-8 (kindle)

Disclaimer:
The material in this book is provided for information purposes only. The experiences discussed in this book may not necessarily be the same as the reader's experience. The reader should consult with his or her personal legal, financial and other advisors before utilising the information contained in this book. The author and the publisher assume no responsibility for any damages or losses incurred during or as a result of following this information.

YOGA FOR MEN

REAL
MEN DO
DOWNWARD
DOG

Greg Cawley

— Learning to bend so you don't break —

Don't turn the page until you read this one!

Here's your quick and very manly style cheat sheet for using this book.

For those of you who might want to skip through parts of this book, I'm going to make it really easy for you. Here's a quick look at what each part is about so you can pick and choose if you want to. After all, we're blokes and some of us don't think we have time for that much reading, and that brings me to my next very important point (after 'yoga IS for blokes!'), and that is, I believe the old saying that 'if you don't have time for an hour of yoga, you need to do two!

Part 1:

The first few chapters are my story, leading into how and why I took up yoga. No dramas, tears, or tantrums, I promise, but they were a challenging few years, and maybe you can relate to having some of those too.

Part 2:

This is about what I've discovered about yoga, and how it was originally developed, mostly for men, as a philosophy and then a way of training for battle. It's also about what yoga actually is. Honestly, most of us, when first faced with the idea of yoga, think it's something a lot different than the reality – so my mission is to demystify yoga for blokes.

Part 3:

Finally, I want to tackle some of the fears we have as men, how we process these, and what we can do for ourselves – the gifts we can give ourselves, and our sons and daughters – by learning to slow down, breathe and be present in each day as it unfolds.

Feel free to skim through any parts but please, even if you are the impatient type who likes to just get the info and then move on, do yourself a huge favour and put aside a couple of hours to dive in and enjoy this book. You'll be glad you did. Truly!

Contents

PART 3

Introduction

Hello, and a big thank you for picking up this book. I really hope you find it to be informative and enjoyable.

But before we go any further, I'd just like to be very clear about one thing ...

Yoga is definitely for men!

We all know that yoga in the today's world is largely practiced by women and all of the media, images and advertising for yoga focuses on the female of the species. I'll cover this aspect of things in a later chapter, but for now let's look very briefly at a bit of history.

- Would it surprise you to learn that yoga was developed and practiced in the early days almost exclusively by men?
- Did you know that one of the first books ever

written about yoga, the *Yoga Sutras* was written by a guy named Patanjali?

- Did you know that yoga was first introduced to the West by a bloke called Swami Vivekananda?
- Would you be surprised to learn that yoga was practiced in the early days by warriors to help them prepare for battle?

Think about the pose Warrior II.

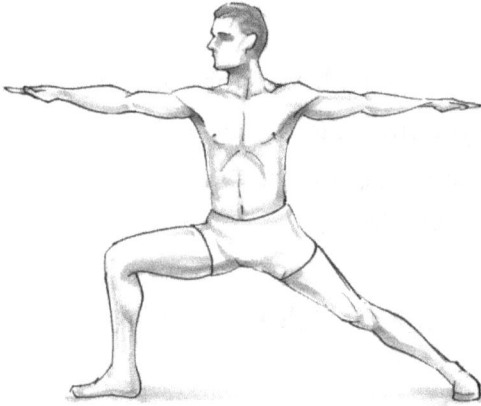

This pose is a representation of the great warrior Virabhadra. The stance depicts him looking down the front arm with intense concentration, eying off the enemy. The back arm is extended, holding his spear. He is holding the spear ready for battle. His mind is intensely focused on what is before him; his body is strong, primed and ready for whatever is coming. This couldn't be more masculine!

This is pretty much how I would describe a yoga class: *concentration, single focus, quiet mind, body strong and ready to move.*

So now (hopefully) we are clear … yoga IS for blokes!

More about this book …

The book is about yoga for men, but it's also about my story through my 60 years of life to where I am now a yoga business owner and instructor.

My name is Greg Cawley. I weigh around 90kgs, I'm built like a brick, I'm going grey and I turned 60 in December 2020. I'm also a Kiwi (New Zealander) now living and teaching yoga to men in Toowoomba, Australia, a large regional town situated due west from Brisbane. How I ended up here and why I started teaching yoga to men is covered in my story.

This book was born from my desire to detail my personal journey and to show that ordinary, everyday guys can practice yoga. And that by doing so, they have the opportunity to really change their lives – mentally, physically and spiritually – for the better.

I was blessed to have enjoyed a very normal and traditional New Zealand upbringing where I was always outside with mates, having fun and exploring. I was always very active and involved with sports when I was younger.

I played serious soccer up to my 30s, I've pumped weights, I've been a MAMIL (a middle-aged man in Lycra, AKA one of those older guys who rides an expensive road bike with a bunch of other MAMILs, and have even at times been found sitting around drinking coffee in cafes in sweaty Lycra cycle shorts). I've walked three marathons, trekked to Everest Base Camp, and I once sweated my way to the top of a 6000m peak in Nepal.

I have been married and divorced and feel very blessed to have my two children, Hanan and Livia, in my life. They are both now in their 20s and are living the Kiwi dream of living on the Gold Coast.

When I left school, I studied for my accounting qualification (ACA) and I started my working life as a chartered accountant. After a few career twists and turns, my wife and I eventually became the owners of manufacturing businesses (this lasted for over 20 years) and at one point we employed 32 staff.

One of my great loves is travel and having new experiences. Having travelled extensively over the years, I've lived and worked in New Zealand, Australia, England, Papua New Guinea and Nauru. My favourite country of all is Nepal (more about that later).

There were times in my business career when I was very successful and made some really good money, but there were also times when things didn't go well. I have been severely depressed and stressed. I nearly lost everything as a result of poor decision making, depression, ego, the global financial crisis and a divorce.

Hopefully my story will resonate with you and you will see I have followed a fairly well-worn path. Pretty normal, huh?

Well, yes, but what isn't totally standard for many blokes is that in my mid 50s, I totally changed my direction and decided to train as a yoga teacher. I have since set up my own yoga business, BrikMan Yoga. *Yoga exclusively for men.*

The tagline for my business says it all:

'No Sheilas, No Lycra, Just Blokes'.

I didn't walk into my first yoga class until I was 49 years of age and I didn't start to teach yoga until I was well into my 50s. It just goes to show that it's never too late. For anything! I'm not particularly flexible, I eat meat and I love a beer or a glass of wine.

The benefits I have experienced from yoga have been immense and I haven't looked back. *You could say that I'm not your stereotypical yoga instructor.*

Prior to hitting 50 and my years of crisis, I saw myself as an accountant and a business man and as likely to become a yoga teacher as fly to the moon.

When you imagine a yoga instructor, I bet you will typically picture them as female and hyperflexible. Or if you do think of a male teacher, and that is by far the minority, you might picture them as smaller in stature, hyperflexible, vegans with a man bun. Nothing wrong with that, but it's not me and probably not you either. I know that this is a generalisation but hopefully you get my point.

My promise for you is that, after reading this book, you will realise that yoga is something that you *can* do – as a male, easily, whatever your age. Yes, even YOU.

You will understand some of yoga's background and its benefits for you as a normal male, whatever your age and stage in life. My personal mission is to help start removing a lot of the common objections and misconceptions that we men typically have and that hold us back from walking into a yoga class. Objections, fears, and excuses such as, 'I'm not flexible enough,' 'I can't touch my toes,' 'I don't like walking into a room full of women,' 'I can't meditate well,' and 'yoga is for girls.'

All of these excuses and more are barriers to yoga for any guy and I aim to remove them and make you feel like a newly minted male warrior – confident and eager to try yoga for the first time.

I also will show you the power of yoga and how it can be a positive agent for change in your life by illustrating the huge changes that have occurred in my own life and in my students' lives since taking up this amazing practice.

Welcome along for the ride.

Let's get started,

Greg Cawley

The Life Cycle of a Yoga Class

I thought I'd start with a little tongue-in-cheek tale about the life cycle of a yoga class through the eyes of a new participant. I'm sure most of you fellas reading this are going to have the same fears, anticipations and trepidations that I did the first time I went to a yoga class. Let's just get all the fears and worries out right here at the start, before we explore what yoga really *is and why it can be an amazing, life-changing experience for you too.*

It starts with the decision to go. Maybe your spouse has been nagging you to try it, maybe your mate from footy says it's the secret to winning a match, maybe your physio swears it's the only thing that'll cure that dull ache in your back.

You walk up to the studio feeling a little nervous – and

fair enough, a yoga studio is definitely right up there in the unknowns. You open the studio door to a sign that says, 'Please leave your shoes at the door.' You unlace your trainers, set them aside and peel off your socks, slightly sweaty with nerves, before giving your pale, more-hairy-than-they-used-to-be, toes a wiggle. *It'll be pedicures next, not just yoga*, you think.

You look around the studio and first thing you check out is the instructor. Do they look normal or weird; do they look like you or are they completely different? You suss them out and that's the first point of comfort or discomfort. Looking like they have just stepped out of a yoga ad, the instructor is small in stature but obviously strong, and they look totally at home in their expensive yoga gear. You were already nervous, but now you really feel like you don't belong, as you look down at your comfy, well-worn workout gear that doesn't really hide your growing beer belly.

You look around the room. Who else is here? *Those girls over there look like carbon copies of the instructor, I wonder if they'll laugh at an old fart like me … those guys talking to them are pretty wiry and they look like they know what's what. But there's that group over there, they all look like pretty average people. There's even a couple of men and women my age, and they don't look too flexible … And that guy there, he looks pretty big, should he even be here?*

You're surprised about the mix of bodies and ages in the

class, and start to feel slightly less nervous – maybe you'll be able to fit in without too much attention. You figure it's still safest to stay at the back of the class where no one can see you. Everyone else seems to have bought their own yoga mat though, so you feel a little self-conscious as you pick one from the studio's pile of communal mats – as if it wasn't obvious enough that you didn't know what you were doing! The communal yoga mats smell faintly of old sweat and disinfectant, but they'll have to do – you take yours and scurry over to a quiet spot in the corner.

The class starts and the instructor starts leading poses; at least they don't seem too complicated. You are constantly looking up to make sure that you are moving correctly. You wouldn't want to find yourself sitting while everyone else is standing! *Crikey, even getting my left and right correct can be a problem!*

Despite being told not to take notice of the others in the class, you are constantly looking around, assessing and comparing. *I think I'm better at this pose than that guy! He looks like he's struggling ... This feels good, feels challenging, maybe I can do this ...*

The class continues, the poses become more difficult and seem to last way too long. *You want me to put my leg where? Get real! Bugger this. I'm not cut out for this stuff!*

This instructor is really starting to annoy you! The agony continues ... *I hate this, I'm definitely not cut out for yoga. What was I thinking?* Trying to keep up. Trying to survive. You feel like you have never sweated so much in your life. *No one told me it was going to be this hard!* How long to go? *I'm dying here!*

The class starts to slow down, and the instructor says it's time for the rest pose. *Okay, this I can do!* Lying on your back, still sweating so much you think you'll leave a puddle, you slowly start to feel every muscle in your body relax and you suddenly realise that you feel good! That pain in your back that you've had for ages feels like it's gone, and you haven't thought about the argument you had with your boss since the class started. You realise that you're loving this moment, even if it feels a bit strange – the squishy mat underneath you, hearing the steady breathing of the other students nearby. You wonder if anyone's fallen asleep in this pose; it'd be easy to. *As long as it's not me, as long as I don't start snoring!*

The class finishes. You pack up quickly, nodding a polite goodbye to the instructor and you're out of there before anyone starts to talk to you. Driving home, you realise your body is tingling, and you are feeling energised.

You were nervous. You were like a fish out of water, but you got through it and it felt great.

That was awesome.
I bloody love yoga!

PART 1

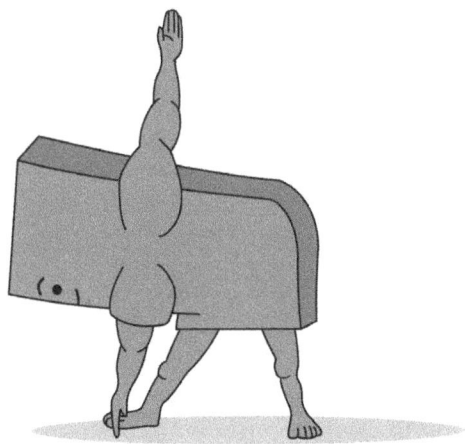

1

My Story

I was born in Wanganui, New Zealand at the very start of the 1960s. Dad worked for the government and mum looked after the kids and the home. My two siblings, Chris and Gail, are ten and nine years older than me so you could conclude that I wasn't planned, and I grew up pretty much as an only child as the others both left home in their mid-teens.

During my early years I lived an active life, mainly spent outside in nature, running around exploring; and like most youngsters back then, I played a lot of sports. I was probably above average ability in most things I turned my hand to, but my passion was with athletics and football (soccer). In both sports, I played at representative levels. It wasn't until my mid-teens when I started to take a keen interest in girls and beer that I gave away the athletics. Football remained a big part of my life right into my 30s and I carried the lessons learned on and off the field through to my later marriage and businesses.

I was keen on becoming a dentist until I discovered I had a severe weakness and basic disinterest in science subjects. My accounting teacher at school pushed me in that direction, but to be honest it never really spun my wheels, and I wasn't particularly good at it. I think probably the thought of making money was the motivating factor. However, I'd pay for that money focus in later life, as you will see!

I studied for my accountancy qualification initially part-time and then with a mix of full-time and part-time years. I wasn't a great student, and was way too interested in extracurricular activities and playing football. I was, of course, lucky enough to have been studying in the years where tertiary study was essentially free and I'm really grateful for that. I really feel for the young people of today who leave university with massive student loans – what a negative start to your career.

My first real job was in chartered accountancy and it was ok. I learned heaps about business and auditing but it never really ignited me. Nothing really did until many years later when I discovered yoga. At the end of my first year of work I travelled to Nauru for a holiday. It may have been an unusual place to go, but my brother Chris was living and working there and I took the opportunity to travel overseas for the first time. I arrived in Nauru on my 21st birthday, 19 December 1981 – and what a game changer that proved to be.

To give the Nauru thing some context, at that time, 1981/82, Nauru was the richest country per capita in the world due to its deposits of mineral rich phosphate that were mined and exported around the world. There were no taxes and it was full of expats – Kiwis, Aussies, English, Irish – having a whale of a time earning tax-free dollars and drinking the cheapest alcohol in the world. It cost $1.29 for a 700ml bottle of Puerto Rican rum, or 30c for a can of Foster's beer. A $2 coin in the pocket would see six cans of Foster's consumed at the staff club on a Friday night – as a starter! To top it off, Nauru at that time had its own airline and a fleet of planes, and these planes were crewed by a multitude of Pacific Islands air hostesses, all single and gorgeous; all looking for fun.

Even though I was only visiting my brother and on holiday, I thought I was in Shangri-La! Cheap booze, beautiful weather, lots of single, available females – yippee! At a barbeque one night just before my holiday ended, I was talking with the manager of the Nauru branch of Barclays bank (the local tax haven), and when he found out I was a trainee accountant, he offered me a position as an accountant/administrator. I was enjoying my time in Nauru so much that it took me about two seconds to decide, 'Yes, I'm going to take this job.' The position was appealing, with its tax-free income – a lot more than I was making in NZ – free housing plus flights. Resigning from my job back home was easy, and two weeks later I commenced my two-year contract in Nauru.

The job was moderately interesting and challenging but it was not my main focus. I played football with the local Solomon Island team (I was the only non-Pacific Islander player) and I learned to play Aussie rules (Nauru's national sport) – but I quickly learned not to get caught with the ball, because a crushed coral pitch with no grass covering and human skin don't mix well. I was living alone for the first time in my life and having a whale of a time – playing football, boozing, scuba diving and chasing air hostesses. I was twenty-one years old and living every young man's dream on a tropical island. I have always described that year as probably the best year of my life. It was a blast!

I was studying part-time by correspondence that year but the New Zealand Society of Accountants decided to change the entrance requirements for my ACA qualification, so I realised I had to leave to go back to New Zealand after that first year ended. I was disappointed, but in hindsight 12 months of solid partying was enough.

I headed back to NZ in January 1983, where I resumed

my full-time study and played football at my local football club again. When I first walked back into the club rooms, the guys who hadn't seen me for a year were quite shocked to see that I had put a lot of weight on – I'd enjoyed too much of the good island life and cheap alcohol. They immediately nicknamed me 'Fatman', a name that has stuck ever since. Up to that point, I had never really had an issue with self-image or my weight. But that nickname changed things. Even though I quickly lost the weight and got into great condition again, the name stuck and so did my concern regarding my weight. To be honest, I'm still really conscious of it to this day. It's interesting (and worrying) how small, seemingly innocent things can affect us emotionally, and how they can carry through our lives – a good lesson to be careful what you say to others.

After my final year of full-time study, I secured a job in the audit division of Deloitte in Hamilton. It was a good job, but, as I said, chartered accountancy never really spun my wheels. I stayed with the firm for a couple of years. In the meantime, I continued playing senior first team football until the club received major sponsorship and employed a full-time professional coach. With the sponsorship they also bought in some very good semi-professional players from the UK, and most of us local guys were pretty much relegated to reserves.

Right throughout my sporting career, and particularly throughout those few years, I had a lot of injuries – ankles, knees, hamstrings and Achilles tendon strains – which kept me on the sideline a lot. I might add that, with yoga in mind nowadays, I can't remember us ever doing any stretching before or after any game – with the exception of stretching to reach over the guy next to me in the changing rooms to grab another beer! It just wasn't a thing back then.

Losing my place in the first team meant that I started playing in the reserves. We had a pretty handy team (full of ex-first team local boys) and won almost every game over a number of years. We were ultra-competitive and had exceptionally high standards, which often meant arguments and a reasonably well-developed bullying culture within the team. If you weren't tough enough to be in that team you were spat out. There was a 'no prisoners' policy and although that meant on-field success, it was, in retrospect, a really horrible environment. I can still remember some players who came into the fold full of enthusiasm and spirit, but left defeated and deflated. Even when we were winning, we were arguing and cutting each other down. You had to be tough to be in that team. It wasn't till later years that I had cause to reflect on this and how it had shaped my behaviour. I had learned to equate success with this 'no prisoners', almost violent, approach to others; really not good. It was very humbling when I came to this realisation and I regret my behaviour to this day.

2

Back to Island Life

In August 1985, I secured a 6-month contract to travel to Papua New Guinea (PNG) to work for the Electricity Commission in Port Moresby. I left for New Guinea in November 1985 – the problem was, I had only just met my wife-to-be, Andrea. Fortunately, while I was in PNG, she travelled up for a couple of weeks and I asked her to marry me.

The original plan had been to travel on my own to the UK and Europe after the end of my contract. But now that suddenly 'me' was a 'we', we decided to return to Hamilton at the end of the contract to get married, work, and save a bit of travelling money. Andrea and I were married in April 1987, and the April after that we commenced our journey to London. We did the usual things that Kiwis did in London in those days. We slept on the floor of crowded flats in Shepherd's Bush, drank too much, partied like crazy and had an amazing time.

I quickly secured work with the Otis Elevator Company in their London head office, where part of my brief was to design and implement a new accounts payable system for the UK. This required a lot of travel around the country to train the branches how to use this system. It turned out that my system was widely condemned by branch managers as being unworkable. However, my young ego was a little in the way of any feedback and I thought it was a perfect solution and couldn't be told otherwise. The system *was* very good technically, but from a practicality standpoint the operators found it to be a nightmare. I only really came to realise that a few years later when I moved into operating my own manufacturing business – so much for accountants knowing everything about running a business.

After my contract ended in London, we travelled extensively through Europe and Asia, spending time in Israel, Egypt and Turkey, before deciding to settle in Brisbane, Australia in September 1989. Andrea and I both got good jobs and I was playing senior football again. Sadly, my continued run of injuries soon ended my high aspirations.

In truth, living in Brisbane and Australia never really suited either of us at that time, so during a visit by Andrea's parents, we expressed an intention to return to NZ and asked if they could keep an eye open for a business in Tauranga. Hey presto, two weeks later we get the phone call – *We have found the perfect business for you!*

We flew back to NZ to have a look at the operation and quickly decided to take it on. It was a pretty easy decision overall, based on two conditions – the business had to be making a certain amount of money, and it was something that I could actually do (you might notice that there was nothing about enjoyment or passion in my requirement for a business, and I paid dearly for that in later life).

We had bought a garage door manufacturing and installation business, Bay of Plenty Garage Doors. I barely knew what a garage door was at that time!

Back to Australia we went to resign from our jobs and pack up our lives, and we were back in NZ only two weeks later, working in the new business and learning like crazy. We took the business over on 1 November 1991. That date is etched in my memory.

Every theoretical decision I had previously made as an accountant disappeared out the window. Very humbling. I knew *nothing* about the practical aspects of running my own operation. It was a huge learning curve, but I was learning fast. Taking over a manufacturing business in November that aligns with the building industry was great timing, as it's a very busy time for business – and for making money. But the pressure is really intense to get everything made and installed before the Christmas close down when everyone goes on holiday for two or three weeks. This Christmas rush is the same every year in building.

To make things worse, the company's garage door assembler didn't take to the idea of a new boss, and quit in late November. I was immediately thrust into not only managing the place and learning 'Business 101' as I went, but I also had to learn how to assemble tilt doors. Anyone who knows me will tell you I'm really not that practical or good with my hands, so this was a big deal.

I would learn the administration and run the business during the day, and at 5pm I would start assembling the doors for the next day, normally finishing at midnight. This was a frigging nightmare and I really hated it, but the silver lining was that I learned the business really well and could tell a good job from a poor one. It was the best thing that could have happened and I know I would never have gone near the factory otherwise and I would have paid for it in the end.

What a great lesson for anyone taking over a new business: start at the bottom and learn from the floor up. You will never regret that. You may not necessarily like it but your knowledge will increase exponentially very quickly and it's also likely to give you real kudos with your new employees. These little things that happened early on really set us up for success and we enjoyed eight really good years of trading. We also won numerous franchise awards, doubled turnover and made great money.

It wasn't all beer and skittles though. You see, we bought the business by borrowing all of the money from Andrea's parents. Her dad was a successful businessman and he was only too happy to lend us the funds to get us going. I'm forever grateful to my father-in-law for having the faith in me and lending us the cash. I know he saw something in me that I didn't. He was very clear with his affirmative answer when I asked him if he thought I could run the new business successfully. This show of faith has been a great lesson for me and I have really tried to apply the same with my own kids.

Andrea, who had come from an entrepreneurial family, always had the view she would have her own business one day. I came from a public servant family and only ever imagined getting a good job as an employee. So, when we came to own our operation and borrowed all of that cash from her dad, things started to go wrong for me.

I felt intense pressure to repay the loan and step up to the level of faith shown in me, and became hellbent on getting him repaid as quickly as I could. I was obsessed and threw every ounce of time and energy into the business. It was my baby. I was driven and from my macho style of life and upbringing so far, I was angry and hard work to be around. That meant I was super aggressive in business and had a 'take no prisoners, suffer no fools' approach to it. I also took an adversarial approach to my opposition which maybe worked initially, but in the end was counterproductive. I used to call business 'warfare', but I have come to realise that no one is a winner in a war.

A business colleague once said to me that you need friends in business. He is so right. Business can be really hard and very lonely and at times you need favours and people or fellow businesses that you can lean on. I wouldn't say I learned this too late, but I can see I paid a price for my initial approach, financially and mentally.

My marriage was, at this time, under a lot of pressure – awful arguments started far too easily and far too often. All I cared about or had focus on was the business. I was stressed and felt constantly under pressure. As always has occurred for me in these situations, I stopped exercising and packed on the weight. This made things worse for me and mentally I was not coping at all well. I have come to realise that when I am in these states, the thing I do the least and the thing I need the most, is exercise. It keeps me in a state of equilibrium and I love the feeling I get in my body when I work it really hard. I thrive off being physical and I suffer badly, mentally and physically, when I don't have it. I now know that exercise is very much a critical part of my maintenance regime.

Andrea and I split briefly for a time, but after a decade

together still had every reason to keep going forward, and when we got back together our son Hanan was conceived and arrived in March 1996. Two years later our daughter Livia came along. Both were absolute blessings and awesome kids, and are now great adults, but the cracks remained in the marriage.

At this point the business was doing great, but I had felt for some time that I wanted to make a change as it had ceased to be a challenge for me. My wife couldn't understand why I would sell it at its peak but that's how it tends to roll with me. I thrive on challenges and get bored easily. It only took a couple of months to sell the business (for a great price) and it also didn't take long for me to come to realise that I was only 38 years old, I needed something else to do, and that the money wasn't going to go far.

I had a few weeks doing nothing in particular and then started looking for another business to buy. We ended up buying a shower manufacturing business called Shower Systems. It was not too dissimilar to the garage door operation in how it ran but it included a wholesaling arm, which I hadn't experienced before, and it had also a poorly run installation arm which I felt I could improve. In my normal do-or-die fashion, I threw myself into it 300%, pretty much ignoring the requirements of my family and marriage. I got the installation arm humming and we encountered pretty good growth over the next couple of years.

However, it quickly ceased to be challenging for me so I started looking at my options again. After looking for a while, we found that a complimentary operation, Rylock Aluminium Windows, a window manufacturing and installation business, was for sale.

I could see how we could put both operations under one roof, save on rent and staffing, and grow both operations as complimentary businesses. This was a great opportunity, but in hindsight this move was the beginning of the end for me as a business owner. Over the years in the building industry, I had often observed full house lots of windows, from various companies, being loaded back onto trucks on building sites to be returned to the factories due to different errors or problems. I clearly remember saying to myself, 'I'm never going to get into that business as it just seems like a nightmare.'

I so wish I had listened to myself. It was! I ended up with a tiger by the tail.

3

The Beginning of the End

The window business was run down when we took it over, but a lot of hard work, the application of success principles that I had learned in the other ventures I'd undertaken along with my accounting background, coupled with a bit of luck and timing with the economy turning upwards, meant that it came into profit very quickly. In hindsight this was actually a real problem, as I had never properly got to grips with how the window business ran. It was a complicated beast.

Both operations, the shower business and the window business, were flying. We were making more money than

I ever hoped for and it seemed way too easy to me. Extra staff were bought on. This included intermediary managers which meant I quickly lost hands-on control and the business got sloppy. On reflection, I'm a good operator when I can maintain hands-on control but I'm not great at working through managers.

My ego had got away on me once again, and I had grown my operations to the size where I could no longer control them. A beachside holiday home was purchased, we were taking prolonged and expensive overseas holidays and our debt burden started to grow.

As a little side note, in 2006 I did take the time to head off to Nepal by myself to trek to Everest Base Camp. This was an amazing experience and was a catalyst for me to start thinking that there must be more to life than working hard and making money. The people of Nepal showed me that you can have happiness and contentment without material possessions. It was very humbling. But I digress ...

I had received some advice years earlier when I was starting out in business which was to 'stay mentally poor'. That means to stay, mentally, in the space where you haven't achieved anything yet and have no spare cash. That way you can avoid the trap of the ego taking over and the expenditure outstripping income. This is great advice and I lived by this for many years, and also observed the failure of many business owners who didn't. It was when I started to forget this advice that things started to go pear shaped.

The earlier large profits and relative ease in making them hid the inefficiencies, and the many overpaid, incompetent staff could hide in the shadows. My own poor decision making was also hidden to some degree. If all you judge your success or failure on is the profit, then there can be a lot going on that you ignore.

It was 2008/2009 when the global financial crisis (GFC) hit, and the shit hit the fan. By that stage we employed 32 staff. Our debt was high and I had lost control as I'd stepped away from the coalface. My marriage was in poor shape but this was also masked up to that point, as everything else was going well and we had a lot of financial freedom.

I can clearly remember coming back to the business after an overseas conference in October 2009 and saw that the order book was drying up. It was clear something was happening and the economy was slowing rapidly. By the time we got to March 2010, we were totally in the shit, both personally and from a business perspective. I had moved almost permanently into the spare bedroom. I was forced to lay off half of the staff, and the businesses were still going south. The window business was dragging the still profitable shower business over a cliff; it was haemorrhaging money and felt totally out of control. Wrong people were doing the wrong jobs, and I was unable to readily change this as I had never really got to grips with the operation and how to run it. The earlier success had masked this as well. My account at the bank was taken to Auckland to be managed by some faceless fish head who hammered me weekly on cash flow and results. They were concerned about their debt and our ability to service it. Fair enough; the debt level at that time was climbing over the $800,000 mark (as I recall) and we were struggling to service it. I would have been worried as well!

I was very unhappy, and even had suicidal thoughts at times as I was in despair at not knowing how to turn this around … oh and my ego was severely dented. Failure was new to me and I didn't know how to react. I stopped exercising. I was spiralling out of control!

4

When Crisis Hits Us

I can clearly remember the moment like it was yesterday.

It was March 2010. I was up in my office at my desk, with my head in my hands and feeling totally defeated, lost and desperate. The window business was hemorrhaging money and was pulling the otherwise still profitable shower business into the pit with it.

I had tried everything I could to turn the ship around. We had cut staff, sold vehicles and looked at and reduced every overhead cost. We had bi-weekly meetings with senior staff to get their input as to how to improve things. Managers were made redundant and more workload and pressure came naturally back onto my shoulders as the owner.

Into my office, unannounced, came Graeme. He was a friend that I hadn't seen for some time, and someone who I had always admired and looked up to as a person and a businessman. Since we last saw each other, Graeme had become involved in a business called Second Base. Second Base had been set up by a former high-flying corporate executive, Zoe Dryden, to take business executives to Nepal for values-based leadership training, and Graeme was working with her in finding suitable candidates. He knew that I had travelled to Nepal before so I guess that is partly why I was on his radar.

We discussed the course, but I was really not in a great space and therefore not too receptive. I was attracted by the prospect of returning to Nepal, but was in a real hole and could not see my way clear to take the two weeks away from the sinking ship – or how to find the money to pay for it. On top of that, I had no idea how I could possibly raise the subject with my wife. Things were really not good between us; communication was difficult and I was sleeping in the spare room.

Graeme pursued me. He could clearly see that I was at a real crossroads in my life: my business and my marriage were both crumbling and I was also in a very poor state mentally. I firmly believe, looking back, that I was within only weeks of a complete breakdown. He called at least once a week for the next three weeks trying to convince me how important it was that I take the step.

I was grateful for his care, but I kept putting him off by using the money excuse.

One week out from the course starting, he called me again.

'I have solved the money issue,' he said. 'You really need to come. You are at a real turning point.'

Graeme had had discussions with Zoe about the state I was in and my need for what the course offered, and she had agreed to slash the course cost by a significant amount. He had removed the money objection and that, along with his concern for me and my trust in his opinion, made it easy for me to say yes. Something in me instinctively told me I *had* to go.

It was a difficult conversation with my wife, I can tell you, but I'm glad I picked up my nuts and explained to her the reasons as to why I needed to go (even though I wasn't totally clear myself, really). I'm also really grateful that she agreed, as my being away required more business time and input from her, and of course she was feeling the overall pressure and desperation as much as I was. I can recall many times sitting with her in my office, with me in tears, totally lost and without the answers I needed to get the business to turn back around.

A week later, in mid-April 2010, I was on a Thai Airways flight to Kathmandu. The first time I landed in Kathmandu (a few years prior when I trekked to Everest Base Camp) it was so exciting to walk onto the tarmac of such a mystical place – one that I had heard about for years and never expected to visit. This time the excitement felt different. I was on a mission but I didn't know what to. I was there on faith.

As we drove away from the airport, I was very calm. I really felt then (as I have when I have visited since) that I had come home. Nepal has a very grounding effect on me; a peaceful effect that contrasts with the chaos of Kathmandu. It's a dirty, dusty, grimy city, mesmerising in its own myriad of fragrances. The roads are overcrowded and full of potholes. There are pretty much no road rules but also very few accidents and no road rage. Cows walk freely through the streets; the powerlines hang above the street in huge clumps like spaghetti in a bowl. A friend who was on the course with me once described the drive from the airport to the hotel as entering a post-apocalyptic *Mad Max* type world. He is not far wrong with that description. But the people are kind, gentle, very welcoming and above all, despite having very little, they are extremely happy and content.

I absolutely love it and felt a deep relief to be back!

5

Discovering Yoga

The course started pretty much immediately on arrival. I dropped my bags into my room and went to the meeting area to join the group. From memory there were seven participants, all from different backgrounds and with differing reasons for being there.

I clearly remember introducing myself but feeling out of place and inferior. I was really in a bad state and my self-esteem was at a real low. I was also really unhappy, and the contrast of me to the others was (I thought) pretty noticeable at the time. I don't recall being told before I agreed to go that yoga would be involved, but on the first morning we all met on the hotel roof at 6am for a yoga session. I normally would have resisted the idea, even made fun of it, but at that point it didn't matter to me. I was up for anything that might improve my present situation. I would *even* try yoga!

Of course, I knew what yoga was about (in a broad sense) but I had never been interested in trying it. It was pretty easy to sit down on the mat for the first time because of the setting: a roof top overlooking Kathmandu at sunrise … awesome! I remember laying on the mat and listening to the sounds of the city. Honking horns, talking, yelling, Nepali music drifting to us on the gentle breeze from the Himalayas, plus the beautiful devotional music that Zoe was playing in the class. The music was sung by a well-known singer, Snatam Kaur, and in the Sanskrit language. It really struck me and felt calming, and connected with me; I had never heard music like that before and I really loved it. I still play it in some of my classes today.

I don't honestly remember a lot about that first yoga class except I was really out of my depth. I was in poor physical shape and overweight as, due to stress, I had completely ceased exercising. I had difficulty in just about every pose; I was lacking in strength and was not at all flexible. Zoe took the class and is a very good instructor, so I imagine that first class was at a reasonably easy level to accommodate all of the participants. Whatever level it was, it was hard for me, but I found myself really liking it for that reason. Physically, I love a challenge and that, plus the music and the peacefulness of it all, had me hooked immediately.

We left Kathmandu and travelled down to a small village near Chitwan on the lowlands near India, where we were billeted with local people and undertook a project with the locals to improve the drainage in their rice fields. We would have a yoga class each morning at sunrise. The venue this time was a small mud-walled school building with a dusty and dirty concrete floor. I didn't miss a class, no matter how physically challenging I would find them, and I really loved the calm I felt lying there, listening to the sounds of the village and the beautiful music that Zoe was playing.

We spent four nights at the village and then went on a four-day trek in the Annapurna range. As there was no hall to practice in, each afternoon after we had finished our walking for the day, we would settle in for an outdoor yoga class, with the 8000m peaks, cool mountain air, and beautiful music surrounding us. What a setting!

I remember clearly one particular afternoon when we were on our yoga mats in a field near Machapuchare (Fishtail Mountain). This mountain is sacred to the Nepalese and as such the summit has never been climbed. We sat there in silence, cross-legged and eyes closed in a meditation. It was late afternoon and the clouds were rolling in along with some distant rumbling thunder. I am still struck by the vivid memory of how I felt right then.

The yoga had really bought me, for the first time possibly in my life into the present moment. The only place where life exists.

Had I not gone through the process of previous yoga classes on that trip, I highly doubt whether I would have allowed myself to become quiet and present enough to fully appreciate the magnificence of what I was experiencing.

I was hooked.

6

Coming Home with a Plan

As part of the course, there was daily one-to-one coaching time with Zoe. The most profound of these meetings for me was in the village near Chitwan, in a mud-walled room of one of the local villager's homes. We discussed why I was there, where my life was at and what I was needing. We had already had a brief phone consultation before the course, so she had some background understanding of me and my plight, and I told her again how much I really hated the window business and was struggling so hard to bring it under control.

She looked at me calmly with gentle but firm eyes, and

simply said (and I still remember it like yesterday), 'Why don't you do your staff a big favour and get out of it? They know and can feel that you don't want to be there.'

What? Wasn't I supposed to knuckle down and solve the problem? Wasn't I there to save it? I'd never considered that I could leave. I felt like I was stuck with it. Surely that was my paradigm – I was the successful businessman, the capable accountant, the problem-solver. Apparently not!

What a relief! Like lightbulbs turning on at the switch in my mind, I could suddenly see a solution to get rid of the dead weight around my neck. A plan was hatched during that meeting, and on the way home to NZ, I would flesh it out until I was ready to present it to Andrea. I would put the window business up for sale. The price didn't matter. I knew that the solution was to get rid of it. I had to cut my losses for the first time in my life!

Zoe held my gaze. She expressed to me that she could see I was observing my life but not really participating in living it. I was watching and analysing. Another slap in the face but in hindsight, very true. I was not at all present most of the time. I didn't know how to let go and have fun. All of the years of my upbringing and my own need to maintain control had indeed led to me being an observer rather than a participant. The only way I could ever loosen up was with alcohol.

After realising this, I really worked to start changing my behaviour more during the trip. Ongoing, the yoga and mindfulness has helped me to be much more present than I was, and as a result life has become so much sweeter and more vivid over the past 10+ years.

The meetings I had with Zoe were profound and I was very aware of the positive affect the two weeks in Nepal had on me and on my future. I remember on the final day, just prior to leaving for the airport, I went up to see Zoe and to thank her. As I went to say thank you, I found I suddenly couldn't speak. I was in tears – totally shaken up by a swelling of emotion and gratitude. Knowing that I was on the right track overwhelmed me. The trip was truly life changing. I'm also eternally grateful to Graeme for his care and his persistence, and to Zoe for her generosity, her wisdom and guidance, and to her introduction to yoga.

I still had the not-so-small task of explaining the plan to my wife! I really didn't think she would agree to sell the window operation and I was very anxious when I raised the subject but, surprisingly, she agreed. She could see it for the pig that it was – and the pig was to be killed!

As part of my discussions with Zoe, we'd decided that the staff should be advised of the business sale and the reasons for it. They knew I wasn't engaged with the business and they sure knew we were in trouble. Now, without Zoe's advice I would have kept the sale really quiet so as to avoid disruption and ensure continuity – but that just would have created additional stress and fear for me, particularly when the staff inevitably got wind of it at some stage. Great advice, I have to say. It made the whole process more honest and they bought into it. I suspect they were just happy that they would eventually get a new boss.

The business was prepped for sale and listed in July 2010. It was sold on 31 March 2011 for little more than stock and plant value, but I was delighted to shed that ugly monkey from my back. We were so lucky to get out when we did, but I'm delighted to say that the business has survived and has grown well under the new and focused owners.

We were back to the core business of shower manufacturing which I understood. I enjoyed the staff and the clients and I knew how to run it well, and so we started the road back to financial recovery. However, after returning from Nepal it became pretty clear that the marriage was beyond repair, and, like a lot of couples who were struggling during the GFC, we were in no position to change our personal situation due to financial constraints.

With the window operation gone and the financial burdens having been lifted a little, attention was now on the poor state of our relationship. We were pretty much estranged. We were still living under the same roof but I had been sleeping in a separate bedroom for the last 14 months. With a huge amount of fear (of both the unknown and the future), sadness for the failure, and concern for Hanan and Livia, then aged 15 and 13, I ended the marriage in July 2011 and moved out.

I'm pretty sure it was 31 July 2012 when Andrea and I (and the lawyers) finally came to our agreements about property and assets, and I took sole control of the shower business. It was a big moment for us both as she walked away from the business and the income that it provided, and I took on the business that was still in recovery mode in a slow economy, plus I took on all of the business debt which was secured over the house at the beach that I was now living in. So, there were some elements of risk for us both. The lawyers said to me after the meeting to agree the settlement, 'It's generally a good agreement when neither of the parties are overly happy.' An interesting viewpoint and probably true enough.

There was a moment in the process of getting to that point where I seriously questioned my desire to keep the business and at one point, we considered selling it and splitting the proceeds. In reality that would not have been a great idea as the whole economy was depressed and the value would have been rock bottom, plus I had been out of the employment market for some time. Was I even hireable? So, the best option, really, was for me to continue.

The mindset I had was that I was just going to grind and get the business back to good profitability so I could rebuild the value of the operation, and then I could look at my options. In hindsight I believe this was sound thinking and showed I was becoming clearer regarding my direction and priorities. Did the yoga help? Probably.

So, the grind started. It was really just a case of head down and bum up: working away at the basics of the operation each day, keeping customers happy and bonding again with the staff after all of the upheavals of the previous few years. I was at yoga three times a week and using that as my support system.

One thing about turning around a business is that it takes time. The best analogy I can use is when a huge oil tanker turns, it can take tens of kilometres for that to happen and it takes a relatively long time. Businesses are like that as well. You can turn the wheel and make the changes designed to make things better, but then you have to wait and stay the course while it turns. It's a big practise of patience and faith that what you have changed will create a good outcome. There were many times that the patience was tested and I really wondered if I had made the correct decision.

As part of my new mindset, I also set about on some personal healing. The whole upheaval, the split, the GFC – all of that had left me pretty raw and battered. My self-esteem was rock bottom. I remember saying to a friend that I couldn't imagine anyone of the opposite sex being interested in me, plus I had been married for 23 years and the whole dating scene was totally foreign to me. My self-image was at an all-time low and I felt like a fish out of water. Having spoken to other guys coming out of long-term relationships I now understand that this is not at all uncommon. It can be a real shock. Have faith guys, it does get better.

The first self-help thing I did, apart from continuing with yoga, was to attend a personal development course in Melbourne. I really had no idea what it was about but Zoe, who had taught me so much in Nepal, was involved with it and she strongly recommended I attend. I went out on faith, no idea what to expect, but I trusted Zoe and her advice implicitly.

In loose terms, the course was all about challenging how you think and encouraging you to take personal responsibility. There's a lot more to it than that, but that is the gist of it. The initial course I went on was just for a weekend. It blew my mind and really opened me up and challenged me. I finished the weekend feeling more in control of myself than ever before, and a month later I went back to Melbourne for another week to finish the initial stage. Some people don't see the purpose in doing personal development courses like that, but I can't speak highly enough about it as far as how it helped me as a person in that moment. I have no regrets at all.

My son Hanan had moved in with me at that time. He was 17, a young fella, not sure of his direction. He was drifting from job to job and mixing with the wrong crowd, and I could see he was making some bad decisions which made me fear for his future. I knew that the same personal development course could really make a profound difference to him so I managed to encourage (well, bribe) him to attend – I had to arrange the time off with his boss who I knew through business and I paid him to attend. I felt that strongly about it. After initial resistance he found great insights and freedom and for the first time I think he realised his own self-worth. We headed to a second course together in Florida. That is when my life took another unexpected turn.

I was attending that course as a qualified student in support of Hanan. Sitting at the table for new students with him was Michelle, a cute, curly-headed blonde from Toowoomba, Australia. I really loved her calmness and her gentleness and I was instantly attracted to her. We worked together at different times during the week and became close friends. Hanan in the meantime was thriving, growing up and really discovering himself. It was money well spent.

Back at home the business was still turning the corner and I was only able to have the time away due to my amazing second-in-charge, Ross Lovegrove. Ross and I worked together for the best part of 15 years. I'm really grateful that he willingly stepped up when I needed him and I felt very comfortable with him in charge. I get the sense that he knew I needed to do some work on myself as he had witnessed the previous struggles at close hand and he just stepped up to the plate. He and I still get together from time to time and I really value our friendship. He's a really good man!

Michelle and I kept in touch, and over the course of the next four months we each attended some more advanced personal development courses over in Florida (as did Hanan). Over the course of these we became really close and it was clear this was more than just a friendship. This was all well and good, but Michelle lived in Australia and I was in NZ and still had a business to run.

What had become very clear to me since taking back control of the business was that my desire and enthusiasm for it was gone. All of the struggles, the arguments and the upheaval had killed all my enthusiasm stone dead. I just didn't want to be there and I wanted out. I had no idea what I wanted to do but I did know that I no longer wanted to run that shower business.

One thing that I did come to realise through doing all this personal development and self-reflection was that I had never really placed much importance on my own happiness, and now I had come to this discovery I wanted more of it. For the first time my focus changed from business to happiness.

A close friend of mine said to me, 'You have half of your life still to live, you may as well be happy.' I've never forgotten those words and they helped to shape my future direction.

I started to spend a lot of time away from the business and with Michelle. Over the course of 18 months, I shuttled between NZ and Toowoomba regularly. Initially I'd go over for a weekend once every month or two, and that eventually morphed into 10 days a month. I was on a first name basis with Air New Zealand cabin crew! As always, Ross just sorted stuff while I was away. The staff reckoned it ran better with me not there. It probably did: my passion for business was gone, the horse had bolted. I had mentally checked out and I had to get out, for everyone's sake. The money wasn't important to me anymore and I just wanted to take my bruised and battered self away to Australia to recover in peace where no one knew me.

I put the shower business on the market in October 2014. I was totally transparent with the staff and it's my belief that they were probably relieved as they knew it was best for everyone that I move on. In earlier years I would have kept this totally private but I'd learned (through good tuition) that it was better to act with honesty and vulnerability and as such the staff became part of the sale process as well.

Once you list your business on the market, as with a house, it can become very frustrating really quickly. All you want is the conclusion so you can move on. Luckily for me the sale process happened reasonably quickly and the sale settled on 31 March 2015, and you know what, I can't for the life of me remember the sale price! It was a significant sum, and I was really happy with it, but I think that shows how I had changed over the years from being totally money focused to happiness focused.

7

Looking Forward to Every Day

When I sold the business, I essentially just turned my back on it and walked away. It had been my baby and I was for the longest time totally tied to it. I have rarely thought about it since and I miss it like a hole in the head. The money problems, the staff issues and the customer problems – good riddance!

I am immeasurably happier now that I'm doing something that I love even though my income is hugely reduced. Lesson learned.

After the business sold, I tied up the loose ends and moved to Toowoomba on a kind of a trial basis to see how things would go. Leaving the kids behind was very difficult, but they were 16 and 18 now and had gotten to know Michelle and were supportive of the move.

I knew virtually no one in Toowoomba and that suited me fine. Michelle gave me the space to decompress and I didn't bother looking for work, I just relaxed, drank coffee down at the deli, got to know a few people and looked at my options and explored where life could take me.

Initially my instincts started to point me back towards business ownership but I'm really glad that I didn't go down that track. I started, with Michelle's encouragement, to look at different paths. I opened my horizons for the first time ever.

The first out-there thing I did was a 9-month body work course in Zen Thai Shiatsu, which is a mix of Thai massage, Shiatsu and yoga. This involves working with your client on a mat and using your body to move theirs as therapy. You've heard the term 'fish out of water' … well I was on dry land and flapping furiously! Here was me at 54, a businessman and accountant all my life learning this weird modality with a bunch of what I termed then as 'alternative' types – yoga teachers, massage therapists, and crystal healers. To top off the discomfort of being a fish out of water, I had to spend 4 days each month on my knees … agony!

The previous year I had managed to convince Michelle to come back to Nepal with me and to climb Mera Peak. It is a 6400m mountain and although difficult and hard physically due to the altitude it's not a hard technical climb. On the way down we had one particular day when we dropped about 2500m and my knees were completely wrecked. They blew up like balloons. It felt like I had razor blades in my knees every time I walked down or up a step. In all honesty, I really thought my trekking days were over.

This pain went on for months, but a lot of massage from Michelle (she is an awesome massage therapist here in Toowoomba if you are looking for one!) and the time I spent that year on my knees, stretching the muscles and ligaments and tendons in Zen Thai and yoga, helped me heal. By the time I had got through the nine months of working the mat in Zen Thai training, my knees were pretty much back to normal.

I had been ready to concede my mobility. My story proves that it's never too late and persistence pays off. Don't get that knee replacement or shoulder surgery straight away, as there may well be far better alternatives like yoga, massage, or acupuncture.

Right from the time I met Michelle, after she found out I was into yoga and that I was searching for a purpose in life post business, she suggested I should become a yoga teacher and specialise in yoga for guys.

Her thinking on this was that:

a. I don't look like your stereotypical yoga teacher at 95kg and built like a brick shithouse, and I couldn't bend like a yoga teacher should.

b. I'm a pretty typical male and blokey in my persona and I relate well to men of all walks of life.

c. I have walked the walk of many men and can relate to them.

'Well,' I thought, 'that's great Michelle, but I sure as hell can't see me doing that! I'm an accountant and a business-man!' That was my self-image at the time ... and I guess I lost that encounter (but the way things turned out, I think I was really the winner!)

So, all of this was percolating in my mind while I was struggling in the Zen Thai course. Me mainly struggling with my self-image and ego. I was so used to being compe-tent and in charge. It was really humbling.

One day while lying in a yoga class on the course and struggling to turn myself into a pretzel (like everyone else), I came up with the name Brick Man. I'm built like a brick and bend as well as one so that would be the name of my (still not decided on) yoga business. A eureka moment! I left the class and told everyone!

I worked on it a little and refined it to BrikMan Yoga, a play on words with the well-known hot yoga franchise Bikram Yoga. So now I had the name of the business I wasn't convinced I was going to start. Good job!

At the end of the Zen Thai course, I was drawn (with Michelle's encouragement – again) to go to a 10-day medi-tation retreat called Vipassana. Vipassana is a worldwide organisation that holds retreats to enable people to learn meditation. It is 10 days, sequestered away from the rest of the world, no phones, no books to read or paper to write on, and it is a silent retreat! You are there totally with your thoughts. You are encouraged to stay very inward and to not even make eye contact with other participants.

For 10 days you lead the existence of a monk. Now, that can be terrifying for some, but I have since recommended it to many, including my son Hanan. Hanan moved to Australia about 18 months after me. It was his way of breaking away from the poor circle he was mixing in and making a fresh start. He was 20 at the time. The week after he arrived, he agreed to go to Vipassana. He is a real chatterbox and a born salesman and loves talking so this was a real challenge for him; but one that he embraced and found great benefit from. So, if you think you can't be silent for 10 days, that boy of mine proves that you can.

The days start at 4.30am with a group meditation and there are several other set meditation times during the day, either in groups in the hall or alone in your room.

For the first three or four days, all that you learn is to focus on the movement of air in and out of your nostrils when you breathe. This is to help focus and quiet the mind ... supposedly. What I experienced was a roller coaster of emotions and thoughts and a virtual movie of my life running through my brain. I remembered people

I had forgotten. I recalled actual moments and conversations. Good experiences and bad experiences.

What I didn't really experience in the first four odd days was a quiet mind! For God's sake, that's why I was there! Nothing I could do would allow my mind to calm and quieten and it was driving me crazy. The mind was in control and I was its slave. It was playing with me.

On the fifth day I had a meltdown during the afternoon meditation session. I couldn't get quiet and I was getting angry. I stormed out of the room and back to my little bedroom. I sulked. I didn't want to be there one moment longer and maybe if I hadn't handed in my keys on arrival, I may well have left. Many people do leave during the course!

I sulked for a couple of hours and went back into the evening meditation and BOOM, I was on. My mind was quieter. I got brief moments of peace and clarity; nothing earth shattering but some peace. *It was amazing!*

What I have deduced was happening was that the mind was sensing it was losing its control and in a final effort to stay in charge it threw every distraction at me it could and that was why I got so pissed off earlier in the day.

The rest of the course was very rewarding and I walked out on day 10 with the best feeling. I felt in control. I was calm and I knew exactly what I needed to do.

8

I Became a Yoga
Teacher ... For Guys

And that was it. The start of my journey to teach yoga!

I think it had taken me so long to get to the space where I could accept myself as being a yoga teacher as my whole persona and self-image for so many years was that of a business man. I literally had to get out of my own way. It took a while but I eventually got there. I seriously doubt I would have been able to change tack like that had I stayed in Tauranga as my persona there was one of a businessman. By being in Toowoomba I had become free to be anyone that I wanted to be, and I did. I still scratch myself when I consider where I am now to where I was.

A few months after finishing the Vipassana meditation course, I started my Level 1 yoga teacher training, a process that took around 12 months. I was still pretty much a fish out of water but this time it didn't really matter to me as I had a purpose and a vision. I had my WHY.

In all previous business incarnations, I have only really had the almighty dollar as my driving force; I was never really passionate about what I was doing and it was all really a means to an end for me.

For me, teaching yoga to guys is a different kettle of fish. It's about passion, it's about serving another rather than myself and it's about helping men. Not a money focus. Don't get me wrong, money is very important but it's not the god it once was to me.

Once I qualified as a Level 1 teacher, I started my teaching journey by instructing two friends in one of my bedrooms at home. From there, I have hired studios and church halls. I regularly get between 15 and 20 brave guys into my classes, and I have held classes at special events for over 100 people.

I have continued with my training and learning and have even travelled to the USA to train with Noah Maze, a very well-respected teacher. Wow, who would have ever believed that?

My men's classes are growing steadily and I have a clear

vision of where I want to take BrikMan Yoga – not just in Toowoomba, but throughout Australia and New Zealand, too.

I am now fitter and stronger than ever. My mind is (mostly) in a great space and I really feel my purpose in life for the first time ever.

My daughter Livia also moved to Australia in the past few years, and both of my kids are doing great. I have so much to be grateful for.

I look back on the last few years and reflect on all of the major decisions that have led to now. It all started with deciding I had to go to Nepal on the course, then to sell the window business, to end the marriage, to attend personal development courses, to sell my shower business, to move to Australia, to undertake Zen Thai training, to go to Vipassana and finally to train in yoga and then to set up my own yoga business.

What a HUGE turn around in the 10 years of my 50s.

Each decision was difficult in its own way and for different reasons but they had to be made for my life to get better.

Guys, particularly of my age group are conditioned to just hunker down and guts things out. Don't be a wimp! As a result, I think that we often will not make decisions because we go into a state of almost suspended animation. We know things aren't right but its way easier to not make a decision and to put up with the suffering rather than to seek help and look for solutions. Do you want to stay in that stressed state and die young? To some of us that may seem as a blessed relief but I can tell you things can improve if you lift your head above the bunker and look for solutions. I was really fortunate as help sought me out at the right time. I've got to be honest though, I may not have had the strength, will or know-how to get myself out of the hole I was in had that not happened. I am one of the lucky ones.

Often, we will sit in the state of uncertainty and fear of making the wrong move. We will often not make major decisions due to the fear of what we might lose. I say, and I have given this advice many times – *focus on what you have to gain.*

I have gained immeasurably from the difficult decisions I have made. Not one has been easy but all have been worth it. Sometimes, to borrow from the Nike slogan, you just have to do it!

Life is great. Thank you, thank you to all of those who have gently and not so gently helped to steer me on this course, and have encouraged me that I have a purpose to fulfil. I am very grateful to you all.

Most importantly, thank you to Michelle for seeing something in me that I couldn't.

But why go on a journey of self-discovery through yoga? Why did yoga have such a profound effect on me? What's it all about? In the following chapters, I explain the history of yoga and why it is for all blokes – not just me, but ordinary guys just like you.

PART 2

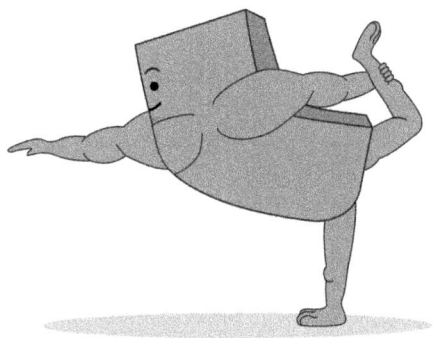

9

Explain Yoga to Me

Yoga has a long and complicated history, and you don't really need to know all the nitty-gritty when you're just starting out. This is a short introduction from how yoga went from an ancient philosophy, to the practice of warriors, to being taught to sweaty students in Lycra.

Ancient origins and battlefields

Most researchers agree that yoga developed in ancient India, but there's a lot of debate about exactly when and where it started. Some think that the origins of yoga stretch back 5000 or even 10,000 years, but it's not until

2500 years ago (500BCE) that we actually see any solid written or archeological evidence of ideas and techniques we'd now recognise as something like yoga in the philosophy of the Sramanas from Northern India. Sramanas were people who believed that they could find their own way to spiritual enlightenment themselves, without the help of any priests or organised religion. They gave up all their worldly goods, left their communities and families, and spent their time on meditation and self-reflection.

These ideas were pretty radical but they were pretty popular, and they were taken up and refined by followers of early Hinduism. One of the first times the word 'yoga' is used in a way we would be familiar with today is in the story *Katha Upanishad* (written in approximately 300BCE), which describes yoga as a type of meditation where a person's senses and mind are bought under control and stilled; as a path to self-knowledge and spiritual freedom. It was around this time that yoga became more of a bloke's activity, as women's freedoms and their role in society became more limited. Yoga developed from here in a society that had strict class and gender divisions, and it was generally thought that spiritual liberation was only possible to men (Hodges, 2007).

The *Bhagavad Gita*, written between 300BCE and 300CE was another big moment for yoga. This epic poem takes place on a battlefield, and a prince is filled with despair about the battle ahead and the choices he has to make, and seeks guidance from a god. The god advises the prince about his duty, responsibility, and spiritual freedom. The story can be seen as a metaphor for our internal battles; that our duty is to fight and overcome the enemies inside us. The *Bhagavad Gita* says that anyone can reach spiritual freedom, and the way to achieve this is through yoga. This is one of the most important early books that talks about the teachings and practice of yoga, and is still often read by people who learn yoga today.

The next important point in yoga history is a book called the *Yoga Sutras*. This is a collection of 196 short statements (*sutras*) about yoga theory and practice which was put together by the sage Patanjali between 325 and 425CE. He collected and organised information about yoga from much older sources and various religious traditions. This was the first time that so much knowledge about yoga had been compiled and organised into one book, and during the middle ages the *Yoga Sutras* was the most translated Indian book. Patanjali defined yoga as having eight key parts – 'eight limbs' – one of which is *asana*, or yoga postures/poses. While this originally meant postures for meditation, the concept was later extended to included more poses, including many of the *asana* we use in yoga classes today.

Different forms of yoga were developing during this time as well, including the famous forms called *tantra* and *hatha*. *Hatha* was based on many of the concepts from Patanjali's *Yoga Sutras*, but included more physical elements that hadn't been seen before. The idea in *hatha* is that it is the mastery of the physical body that leads to enlightenment, so the style included many more physical poses *(asana)* and breathing exercises. By the 1700s, *hatha* had become a popular and predominate form of yoga.

Religious warriors have long been a part of Indian culture, which may seem strange but it's easy to see how soldiers and monks are similar – they both need to be self-disciplined, to be able to survive on limited food rations, to live in hard or uncomfortable conditions, and to respect their leader. Yoga was used by warriors to train and strengthen their bodies ready for battle, and it also allowed them to overcome their fear of death (Pinch, 2006). By the 1700s, yogi warriors were the most common type of warrior in India, numbering in the hundreds of thousands (White, 2012). When the British colonised India in the 18th century, militant yogis 'engaged in exercise regimes to make them tough, in order to oppose the British ... In this period, to be a yogi often meant to train as a guerilla' (Doniger, 2014).

Health and fitness, a big focus of ancient Greeks, had reemerged as an interest in the West from the early 1800s as theories about the physical and moral benefits of exercise became popular. The British took these ideas with them into India, and concepts like gymnastics and body-building started to impact on yoga forms and styles at the same time as traditional Indian culture was being discouraged (Doniger, 2014).

The West, bored housewives, and the Beatles

Western interest in Indian culture and philosophy had started in the mid-1800s, but really took off in 1893 when Swami Vivekananda travelled from India to the United States, and spoke at the 'World's Parliament of Religions' in Chicago. He was really popular with both the crowds and the press, and spent the next two years travelling around the US and the UK, giving lectures and classes on Hinduism, Buddhism, and yoga. His focus was more on the practice and technique of yoga, particularly meditation, rather than the religious elements of it, which may have made him easier for a Western audience to connect with. In 1896, he published *Raja Yoga*, his interpretation of Patanjali's *Yoga Sutras* specifically for a Western audience; the book was an instant success, and has had a huge impact on the understanding of yoga today. Vivekananda's success opened doors for other famous yogis to travel to Western countries, like Sri Yogendra and Swami Paramhansa Yogananda, who both found great success in the US with their own interpretations and styles of yoga from the 1920s onwards.

In 1948, a woman called Indra Devi opened a yoga studio in Hollywood and found great success teaching yoga to movie stars including Eva Gabor, Greta Garbo, Yul Brynner, and Gloria Swanson. Devi had studied with the famous yogi Tirumalai Krishnamacharya in the late 1930s. He didn't want to teach her at first, because he had never taught a woman or a foreigner ever before – but she impressed him so much that he trained her to be a yoga teacher herself, and she became the first Western woman to teach yoga in India. Devi taught her own form of *hatha* yoga, focusing on *asana* and breathing but avoiding too much spirituality. She marketed yoga as a solution to anxiety and the secret to youth and beauty – which made it particularly appealing to women. Indra Devi's style of yoga is one of the really important points when yoga turned from a predominately male activity to the mostly female one we think of today.

Through the 1950s and 1960s, yoga's popularity in the West continued to grow, with its focus on physical health, well-being, and improving body shape and tone. It was still being strongly marketed towards women at this time, emphasising the power of yoga to lose weight, delay aging, and increase beauty (Hodges, 2007). The first yoga studio in Australia was opened in Sydney in 1950 by Michael Volin, who had studied under Indra Devi. The Gita School of Yoga was the first yoga studio in Melbourne, opened by Margit Segesman in 1954.

Television also helped to boost the popularity of yoga in Western countries during these decades, with the first television show about yoga, *Yoga for Health*, produced in America in 1961. The creator, Richard Hittleman, had studied yoga in India and was really interested in the spiritual side of yoga, but focused on the physical, non-spiritual elements of the practice in his TV show. In Australia in 1962, a woman called Roma Blair had a mid-morning television show, *Relaxing with Roma*, designed to introduce yoga to housewives.

The 1950s and 1960s also saw counter cultures take hold in Western countries, as young people rejected social constraints and expectations – especially after the Second World War – and started looking for freedom, peace and spiritual answers. Many of them turned to Eastern philosophy, religions, mysticism, and practices, which included yoga and meditation, for answers. The Beatles had a huge influence on the popularity of Eastern spirituality and practices (not to mention clothes and music) among Western youths when they travelled to Rishikesh in northern India to study with the Maharishi. This received huge media attention around the world, and suddenly everyone wanted to be cool, meditate, and get in touch with themselves just like Ringo was doing! Yoga also appealed to 'women's lib' types in the 1960s, who liked the idea of yoga giving them freedom of movement and dress, a way to express themselves, and connect with their 'inner selves'.

The use of yoga in the search for spiritual enlightenment

continued into the 1970s and 1980s, what we'd call the 'New Age' types – but yoga also continued to grow in popularity as a form of exercise as the fitness industry really began to take off, and also as a therapeutic option to relieve stress, anxiety, or chronic pain alongside traditional Western medical treatments. These ideas continued through the 1990s up to today, but we've also seen yoga becoming a more commercial industry. Now there's not only books, courses, classes, holidays and retreats for yoga, but yoga equipment, accessories, clothing, and even jewellery. The yoga industry has boomed, and is worth at least US$88 *billion* dollars worldwide, with the Australian industry being worth US$716 million[1]. The global worth is estimated to hit a boggling US$216 billion by 2025.

Yoga is big business and there are major worldwide companies and franchises taking advantage of this growth. This industry growth has also seen the types and styles of yoga offered and practiced worldwide boom too. There are fairly 'traditional' styles of yoga like Ashtanga, Iyengar, Vinyasa, Kundalini, and Yin; styles that focus on strength and weight loss like Bikram, Hot, Acro and Power yoga; and styles designed for specific health outcomes like Restorative and Prenatal yoga. We've also seen more

---

1   This is the value of the combined Pilates and yoga industry globally and in Australia, produced by https://www.ibisworld.com/au/industry/pilates-yoga-studios/4198/. Yoga is by far the biggest segment, even though the two fitness areas have been grouped.

'novelty' styles of yoga popping up over the past few years: Beer Yoga (with participants drinking before, during, or after practice), Goat Yoga (yoga done with baby goats running around), Doga (yoga designed to be done with your pet dog), Broga (yoga for 'bros' with cardio and high intensity interval training thrown in), Naked yoga, Hip-Hop yoga, Laughter yoga, Karaoke yoga ... who knows what they'll come up with next!

Different styles of yoga offer people different things, and it can be good to try one of the novelty styles or an online class if you're really nervous about joining in. Don't be scared to try different styles or different teachers until you find one that works for you.

Why has yoga continued to be such a popular activity? It makes sense when you look around at the world we live in – it can be a stressful, worrying place, and we know that it takes a toll on us. We know we need to look after ourselves, both on a physical and mental level. Yoga's great exercise and feels good, but it provides all sorts of refuge.

What does yoga mean, exactly?

The word 'yoga' has a pretty complicated history itself! It originates from the Sanskrit word *yuj*, which can be broadly translated into English as 'to yoke together' or 'to unite'. In ancient Indian texts, the word was originally used to describe a war chariot in its entirety – the chariot itself, the horse or team of horses pulling it, and all the harnesses and straps used to join them together (White, 2012). In particular, it was used to describe divine chariots that gods travelled in, and the divine chariots that would take a warrior killed in battle into heaven. This image continued to develop in ancient Indian poetry and hymns, with priests describing their minds as being 'yoked' to inspiration, which allows their earthly words and their divine message to become one.

It is this idea of the union of the individual with the divine, or a universal consciousness, that we see consistently through the development of yoga in history. What I understand yoga to mean is the unification of different parts of ourselves – our mind, our body, and our spirit – through our yoga practice. We bring all of these elements into one, concentrating on our breath, and by doing this, we become one; whole and complete.

Yoga and yoga philosophy

You might have noticed in the history section that to begin with, yoga was pretty closely tied up with religion, and it had a lot to do with bringing a person closer to god or to enlightenment. But it's also always had a lot to do with how to live your life well, and how to find peace and relief in the world. The philosophy of yoga is really awesome and is very applicable to us as men in the modern world, especially if you can look past a bit of the religious stuff. Yoga is a way of clearing our minds and giving us better focus; it's a way of bringing our minds and bodies into better alignment; it's a way of relieving stress and tension from our minds and our bodies; and it's a way to learn how to not let your bloody ego get in the way!

Yoga's history, including the philosophical stuff, is often interwoven into a class. To a newcomer, this can be a bit confronting or uncomfortable. I'd say it can be akin to having the Bible read to you during a spin class! Don't let this put you off, though – if you're in a class that is going a bit too heavy on the philosophy too quickly, just focus on your breathing and your movements, and let it wash over you.

My personal methodology as a teacher is that, first and foremost, a male yoga class needs to get moving, stretching, sweating, and working hard. I stay light on the 'woo woo' until I have a good feeling for the class and the guys in it. After a time, I start to add in a few bits of philosophy as it can really add to the experience, and for some guys it can be just what they need to hear to help them in their lives. A bit of philosophy at the right time can really cement them into yoga, because they see how it all works together – the body and the mind.

I'm always a bit surprised (and maybe I shouldn't be) when one of the guys repeats something back to me that I said in a class weeks ago. It always strikes me that when the mind is focused and quiet, that's when the good things can get in.

Get them in, shut their minds up and get them moving. Simple but effective!

64

10

What Does a Yoga Class Look Like?

Yoga classes can vary pretty significantly, depending on the style of yoga, the teacher, and where it's held. Some studios are very small and might only fit five or six yogis, while some classes are held in halls or gyms that might fit 40 or 50. If you do an online class, your studio might be your bedroom or your backyard! Purpose built yoga studios often have a wooden floor, and depending on the style of yoga, might have blocks, cushions, bolsters, straps, and blankets that can be used to help support you in poses or help to get you deeper into a pose.

Yoga is always practised barefoot, and almost always

using a yoga mat to stand or lie on. Most yoga studios will offer yoga mats for hire or for free use for those who don't own one. In the yoga room, the mats will usually be arranged on the floor, side-by-side, facing the instructor's mat which will be at the front.

With yoga originating in India, the accepted language of the yogi is Sanskrit. In a yoga class, you will often hear the poses being introduced in both Sanskrit and in English. For example, the rest pose at the end of a class, Corpse Pose, is *Savasana,* and Downward Facing Dog is *Adho Mukha Svanasana.*

The format of each class can vary quite a bit too, and how the class will run depends on the style of yoga, the policies of a studio, and individual teachers. A Bikram yoga class, for example, will be run identically wherever you go, with 26 poses and 2 breathing exercises done in the exact same sequence every time during a 90-minute class. This uniformity is a little unusual, but that's Bikram for you. Yoga classes in other styles are not so uniform, and the sequence of poses is chosen by a teacher depending on their goal for the class and the students – the specific poses and their order in a class for relaxation will be different from those in a class to boost energy or strength, for example.

Most classes will end, and sometimes also start with the greeting, '*Namaste.*' If you've travelled in Nepal or India, you will recognise this as a common greeting or farewell.

It literally translates to 'I bow to you', and is usually said while slightly bowing the head and hands together in a prayer-like position in front of the chest. In the sense we're using it in yoga class, it is saying, 'The divine (god) in me recognises the divine (god) in you.' I think it's a lovely way to finish a class; recognising that we're all equal, that we all have something divine within us and it acknowledges us all.

Etiquette and good habits for yoga

Etiquette is another thing that can vary quite a bit between studios, but there are a couple of points that stay pretty consistent between studios.

It's pretty important to arrive on time. Yoga class is the time when you can connect with yourself and recharge, so you don't really want to be rushing around and all stressed out to being with. Arriving on time allows you to find a space, set your mat up, collect any props, and get ready for the class without disturbing anyone else. Some studios can be quite formal and have a policy of complete silence, where you stay silent and bring yourself inward once you enter the studio. In these types of studios, students enter the room and sit or lie on their mat without talking until the teacher arrives. Other classes are a bit more social and informal, and friendly chatting between the teacher or students before and after the class is okay. Make sure to turn off your phone or any other electronics that might interrupt the class, too!

Yoga is always practiced with bare feet, and most studios will ask you to leave your shoes near the entrance of the studio. It's great to be able to feel the mat under your soles, and feel the grip and connection with the mat and the floor underneath. Going barefoot in yoga is also a good opportunity to let the muscles in your feet stretch and get stronger, and can help you feel balanced and more stable. Leaving your shoes at the studio door also means that no mud or muck gets tramped through the place. You spend a lot of time on the floor in yoga, so you want it to be clean!

You'll generally use a yoga mat in your class, and you'll probably want to buy your own. I'd strongly suggest avoiding thick or really spongy mats. While they look like they will be really comfortable, they can actually create a problem when you are in a balancing pose as they mean that you're standing on an unfirm base. I would recommend a compressed mat of 5 or 6mm thickness; but there are thousands of styles of mats out there at a huge range of prices. It's best to talk to your yoga teacher or someone who practices yoga before you go out and buy your own. Whether you buy your own mat or borrow one from your studio, it's good etiquette to keep it clean, to prevent germs from spreading or getting too smelly from sweat. Most studios will have a disinfectant spray ready for students to wipe their mats down with after class, and a gentle scrub with mild soap and water once a month is good for most people.

Yoga fashion has become pretty big business. If the class is not a man-only class, you're likely to encounter a room mostly full of women wearing tight, stretchy Lycra workout gear. You don't have to go out and buy anything special, and you don't have to wear Lycra if you don't want to. For guys, I recommend wearing loose-fitting, breathable clothing. Shorts and a singlet are the best options for me – they just need to be loose enough to allow you to move and stretch freely, especially the shorts around the butt and the thighs, but the singlet needs to be tight enough that it won't fall up around your head in an inverted pose. It's a bit of a balancing act to get this right. But definitely wear underwear. The guy behind you doesn't need to see anything loose and jangly, if you get what I mean!

Yoga, no matter how relaxing, is still a form of exercise, so don't forget to bring a clean towel with you to mop up! You'll also need to have the energy to do it. I would discourage you from eating a full meal or drinking too much water in the two hours before a class, though. Light, healthy snacks are okay, but a lot of poses involve forward bending and twisting, and these are very uncomfortable if you've got a full belly.

What happens in a BrikMan Yoga class?

My studio is a little different from most others. BrikMan yoga classes take place in a hired hall which fits quite a few fellas without anyone feeling crowded. I like to keep it pretty relaxed and informal, and I don't have any set rules about being silent before classes. Once the guys walk in, they are free to either go into their own space and lie down quietly, or they can chat with me or their fellow students (who, quite often, become friends).

My class structure does differ from class to class, depending on the style I'm teaching and sometimes on the audience, but this will give you a general idea of the structure of a 'normal' class I might take my students through.

We begin with everyone sitting cross-legged on their mats, facing the instructor. Some students might be sitting on a yoga block if they have a tight back or hips. I often sit on a block to take the pressure off my knees, hips and back – it's all about working with your body.

The first few minutes of class are about quietening down, bringing the focus inward, connecting to our breath and becoming present. I like to suggest to my students that they concentrate on the movement of air in their nostrils, a technique and image I found particularly useful from my Vipassana meditation course. The breath is really the essential factor in yoga. It connects our movement with our mind. Without our breath and our focus, we'd just be stretching. In yoga we always breathe through the nose.

This helps to quiet the central nervous system and by really focusing on our breath, our mind naturally quiets down too and we get a chance to get out of our minds. One of my little catch phrases for class is, 'men getting out of their minds.' I think that sums it all up.

Breathing through the nose has some other pretty good benefits: it cleans and filters air we take in, improves lung volume, and results in approximately 20% more oxygen absorption than breathing through the mouth. One of the reasons for this breathing through the nose takes more effort, adding 50% more air resistance and also giving your heart and lungs a bit more of a workout (Ruth, 2015).

The initial breathing and meditation are followed by around 10 minutes of warm-up stretching and movements. Following that is the meat of the class, which involves approximately 30 to 40 minutes of vigorous movement and stretching; sometimes holding poses for a few breathes, sometimes (like in a Vinyasa class) moving to another pose after only one or two breaths. This is where the strength kicks in and the sweating starts – it can be hard and challenging.

The final 10 to 15 minutes are for slower stretching and winding down, often in poses lying on our backs, with approximately the last 7 minutes of class being our rest pose, *Savasana* (Corpse Pose). This pose ends all classes. We lie still on our backs and fully relax, closing our eyes and letting our bodies melt into our mats. We breathe deeply and quieten our minds to come to a meditative state.

I often describe this final pose as like the end of a business meeting, where everyone present comes to agreement on what was said and what is to happen going forward. The mind and body unify, becoming quiet and still and we integrate what has happened in the class. Often students find themselves becoming so relaxed and they start to drift off to sleep. It's not uncommon – I've been in classes where we're finishing up *Savasana*, and someone gives out a great big snore!

At the end of the class, we sit up again in a cross-legged position. I give students the option to leave their hands resting on their knees, or put their palms together in front of their heart in a gesture of gratitude – gratitude to themselves for having made the effort to be there and do the required work, and gratitude for all of the other men in the class for having shown up and done the hard work, too. Finally, we farewell each other with *'Namaste'*. Like I said earlier, I think it is a lovely way to finish our practice and acknowledge each other.

After that, some of the lads will chat as they pack up and get ready to go, and some may just lie quietly in their own space for a few minutes while they come back to their bodies after *Savasana*. Different classes vary in intensity and effort, and I often get men who've just experienced their first yoga class come up to me after, expressing how much harder it was than they had expected. It's not tiddlywinks!

Yoga is as old as the hills and as deep as the ocean. Some people devote their whole lives to the study of the craft, its origins and its philosophies. I know it can all be a bit overwhelming for men who are new to yoga, but I say just find a class and a teacher that feels right for you, and get started – concentrate on getting your body moving and feeling comfortable in the class. The rest will come.

PART 3

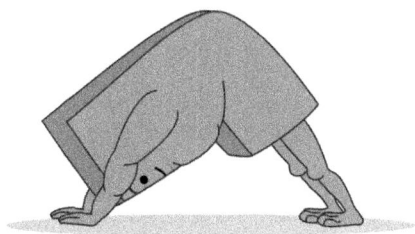

11

Why Guys Don't Do Yoga

Earlier in the book, I talked about some of the times in the history of yoga when it shifted to be more popular with women. But a bit of beauty-industry marketing surely can't override thousands of years of yoga history and the relationship men had with it – so something else must have changed, either in our psyche or in the world. What's the story? Why aren't guys flocking to yoga, when the benefits are so many and so well known?

In my opinion, there's a lot of reasons for this: misunderstandings about what yoga is, societal expectations, and men's self-esteem. If you've read the chapter on the history of yoga, you'll probably already have a good idea about why a lot of people today misunderstand yoga and who it's for, so let's talk a bit about the other two big issues about why guys don't do yoga.

Societal expectations

'Typical' males

Let's face it, fellas, the term 'typical male' has been bandied around since way before Tina Turner made it a big hit in the 1980s! So, what is the paradigm for a 'typical male' in the Western World?

We, particularly men in my age group, were raised to be tough, brave, and independent; we were taught to be powerful, in control, and assertive – even aggressive. The 'boys don't cry', 'man up' kind of attitude. We were raised to believe that our role was to get a good job and work hard at it, to find a good partner, have children, and bring home enough money to provide a good life for them. We were taught that it wasn't right for men to show too much emotion, or be too sensitive. It was how most of our fathers and grandfathers were raised, and it was a pretty natural progression of life to follow back in the mid 20th century.

We were taught to be competitive too, and when it came to sport (again, this is from my baby boomer perspective), we were expected to play team sports. In NZ and Australia, rugby union, rugby league and AFL – 'manly' teams with short shorts and the Canterbury jerseys – were at the top of the hierarchy for many, but rowing, tennis, swimming, cricket, and athletics were pretty popular too. These sports can give us fantastic life lessons, of course, but high intensity impact sports can have a severely negative impact on our physical health and our bodies as we age – especially when we were told to 'tough it out' or 'walk it off' if we got hurt. Even as guys in my generation got older, retired from intense sports and took up cycling, golf, or the gym, the attitude to sports really seems like an extension of the expectation we grow up with as males: work hard, put in the effort, head down bum up, don't give up, win!

For a lot of guys who feel the weight of these expectations (and who don't understand what yoga is), yoga doesn't seem to really fit in: it's not a competitive sport that you can win; the idea of 'getting in touch with yourself' seems a bit sensitive; and so many women do it that it surely can't be the right activity for 'real' men!

Work/Holiday

Men in my generation were also taught that it was important for men to always be in control. Have you ever noticed how difficult and stressful a family holiday can be? I clearly remember one family holiday where me, my wife, and our two kids (both under 5) headed to Noumea to stay at Club Med. We'd specifically chosen Club Med for their famous kids' club – the concept of dropping the kids off for the whole day before sauntering off for a nice relaxing time together was mega appealing!

Well, guess what? The bloody kids wouldn't go to the kids' club! They cried and carried on so much that we just had to keep them with us. There we were, in a tropical paradise but unable to relax and enjoy it, because we had to supervise our two toddlers. There was another couple there, John and Sue, with two kids the same ages as ours and with exactly the same problem. I remembered seeing them checking in beside us at Auckland Airport, and thinking that John looked really on edge and stressed. We spent a lot of that holiday hanging out together, and John ended up confiding in me that he found family holidays really stressful, and he didn't know why that was the case when they were meant to be happy occasions for the family to bond.

In my humble opinion, and coming from someone who totally agreed with John's assessment of family holidays, it's about loss of control for the male.

Most of our time is spent at work. It's an environment where for the most part – depending on our circumstances, of course – we will generally have a degree of control over how and where we spend our days. We choose what we do and when we do it. It's generally predictable and steady and it's where we get a lot of our sense of purpose and self-esteem. It's a *safe place* for us guys and for many guys it fulfills that social expectation of our purpose as a worker and provider. When it comes to going home to the kids, then all bets are off. It's chaos! There's no respect for your personal space or time or agenda. In my day, it was more common for men to go out to work while women stayed home to look after the kids – and once dad got home at the end of the day, mum was just glad that the kids might be off her plate for a little while! Now, of course, both parents in many families go out to work, but that just means that both parents feel the loss of control when they leave their calm workplaces and head home for the day. I adore my kids, but to be honest mostly I'd rather be at work! I hope it's not just me that feels like this.

So, imagine how this is magnified when it comes to the family holiday. There's no work to retreat to and hide in. You're on duty 24 hours a day with the family. You have to be available for the kids, you also need to learn how to operate as a couple in a close environment when you normally have your own space, and often you're still the one in charge of organising the holiday and making sure everyone's having a good time.

I know I'm being a bit controversial here, but I want to point out the different balls that guys have in the air and how difficult they can be to juggle. It's hard for men, and it's definitely hard for women as well, and it is little wonder that separations increase over the Christmas period.

This social expectation that guys should always be in

control can also prevent guys from doing yoga. You can feel pretty out of control when you're trying something new or unfamiliar, and you can feel pretty out of control when you're pushing back against some of those deeply ingrained social expectations.

All of these societal expectations of men, and whether we feel like we are or aren't meeting them, can stop us from doing all kinds of amazing things – like yoga – but they can also be pretty damaging to men's self-esteem.

Self-esteem

I think most of us in our society today are out of balance in how we judge success. Not only do we have those other expectations digging away at our self-esteem, we're hellbent on adhering to the societal expectation that material success is the only thing that matters; thinking that is how our self-esteem is established and grows. Climb the corporate ladder, make more money, buy a fancy car, move to a bigger house in a better neighbourhood, send the kids to a more expensive school – these types of achievements can be pretty great, and, sure, they can help us grow in status and self-esteem, but they can also destroy us if we think that money is the only path to happiness.

Only a small percentage of any population will be able to reach and achieve the highest levels of material success – the top job, the best car, the biggest house. This, of course, means that everyone else will struggle or fail to achieve some or all of the expectations put upon them by society – no matter how hard they try. What I see – and have personally experienced – as a result of this is a mental health crisis for men everywhere.

Guys get to 40, and the pressure is still increasing on them to work harder, to provide more, to stay in great shape, and to find time to be a great husband and father. If society demands this and you can't live up to it, it can really lead to feelings of hopelessness, desperation, and failure.

I, personally, have been on both sides of this fence. I've had a pumped-up ego and high self-esteem from success in sport and business, and I've also been to some very low depths and dark places particularly when my business and marriage started to fail. My self-esteem was through the floor, I became depressed and considered suicide. It is a tragedy that in both NZ and Australia, suicide rates amongst males are some of the highest in the western world. How can this be, when we really do live in two of the best countries in the world when it comes to affluence and quality of life?

We are out of balance, guys!
Thinking that good self-esteem comes from pursuing material achievements and trying to live up to unrealistic expectations only leads to stress, burnout, and misery. With balance comes contentment and happiness.

Kiwis (and I know because I'm one of them) are really bad at having an inferiority complex and believing we have to work twice as hard as anyone else to get ahead and be recognised. Aussies have a slightly more laid-back attitude but overseas we are both sought after employees because of our work ethic. This is NOT always a good thing!

We need to change our idea that success and self-esteem come from money, possessions and winning, to balance, happiness and contentment. We need to embrace new habits which support this, such as yoga, tai-chi and meditation. We need to get better at living a good life. Money need not be our dictator!

The country of Bhutan has a national measurement of its success called the Gross National Happiness (GNH), which is taken just as seriously as economic measures like the Gross Domestic Product. The GNH measures the overall quality of peoples' lives, including things like their psychological wellbeing, community vitality, and how their time is spent. The GNH is designed to ensure that the country's material and spiritual development happen together, and that the citizens' overall wellbeing is equally valued as their economic output. Pretty cool, huh?

We are judged by our success (both by ourselves and others) but our success requires so many different mind-sets and pressures, and quite frankly most of us guys don't have all the necessary tools in our tool belt.

If we focused more on happiness and wellness and less on material success and achievement, I believe we would be in a better space to be better men, better parents and better partners. We need to be more like Bhutan and bring value to this. If we do, then wellness practises like yoga and meditation would become more acceptable and perhaps essential in the pursuit of what is seen as the 'new' success formula.

Men would be more drawn to what helps them achieve the measures of success.

Funny how what we need is not what we value.

Bear in mind that I am a class-A alpha type bloke who lived and breathed this stuff nearly all my life – the high impact team sports, the money-chasing, the need to be in control – but I'm going to let you in on a secret: you don't need to bust a gut, be it at work, at home, or with sport. You don't need to be the best or the toughest. What you really do need is to find balance – balance between what is good for you and what you need to achieve.

12

Why They Should

The last chapter ended up with a bit of a chat about balance being the missing factor for a lot of blokes. I strongly believe that yoga is a powerful tool that men can use to change their view of the world and themselves, build up their self-esteem, and bring balance to their lives.

Calmness

The single most positive impact that yoga has had on me, right from the word go, has been being able to find and maintain a state of calmness.

Even before I understood anything else about yoga, I understood the power of the intense focus on the breath.

Feeling and listening to the tide of your breath rolling in and rolling out can be very transformational and very, *very* calming.

You might have noticed that when you get angry, uncomfortable, or in any heightened state of emotion, your breath shortens and becomes more rapid. Conversely, if you are relaxed and comfortable, your breath will generally be long, slow, and rhythmic. Your breath can be a giveaway to your internal and mental state.

To me, slow and steady breathing helps to create space. In times of stress, it's useful to create space between the stimulus (whatever it is that is stressing you) and your reaction. This space helps to determine the response and the outcome. For example, if someone says something hurtful or annoying to you, an immediate verbal comeback generally isn't going to provide the best outcome – you'll probably say something equally hurtful or angry and it'll just make things worse. By slowing things down and connecting to your breath, breathing deeply and slowly, you can create space between the stimulus (what was said to you) and your response, and that space gives you the chance to consider your response and how to make it – if you make any at all.

Always ask yourself: 'What will happen if I say nothing?'
– Kamand Kojouri

I've certainly learned how to keep my mouth shut rather than instantly reacting to everything, and I've learned how to create that space in myself. Now don't get me wrong, I'm no saint and I still have some shitty outcomes at times when I haven't stayed calm. But I will say that my outcomes are way better than they used to be – simply because I've learned to stay calm by being present and connecting to my breathing.

That might sound pretty simple, but it's not necessarily easy and it takes time and training to control. In yoga, we do two distinct things that help us with calm:

- **We focus on the breath.** The breath we take in yoga is through the nose. Breathing through the nose regulates and slows air flow, and helps to lower blood pressure and stress.
- **We focus on the process,** rather than the outcome. Yoga is all about staying present and concentrating on the action we're doing, rather than the outcome, e.g., getting a pose 'perfect' or holding it for the longest time.

Doing yoga trains you to stay present, breathe deeply and slowly, and let those stressful moments pass.

When the mind is calm, how quickly, how smoothly, how beautifully you will perceive everything.
– Paramhansa Yogananda

Yoga trains you to get into and stay in a mental space where you don't get triggered; where you don't react; where you stay very present and in the moment.

When I work with sports teams, I ask them what even a split-second of calm during an intense game would do for their decision making. Perhaps when you're under pressure at work, you would handle it better. Maybe at home if you have a tense exchange with your partner you might not react and say things that would ordinarily inflame the situation or cause regret. One of my students (you can read his story in the case studies at the end of the book) mentioned that the ability he had found through yoga to just stay calm and breathe had made his home life better.

Imagine the difference that having access to this state would make to you. How would it be for you to use the same techniques that you learn in yoga in your normal life and what a difference could it make to you?

Stay calm inside! You will then see that outside storms of life, even the most terrible ones, will turn into soft winds.
– Mehmet Murat ildan

Clear decision making

In all of our lives there come points in time that we need to make choices and decisions. Hardly ever do these BIG decisions come at a convenient time or are easy to make.

When it comes to making decisions, I will generally weigh up the pros and cons, and I'll nearly always write them down so I can get a visual appreciation of what they are. I'm a visual person, so if you are trying to sell me something, I'll insist on seeing something in writing before I even consider it. A verbal presentation will not suffice for me, it's just how I'm wired.

Despite all of this, a large part of my decision-making process will come down to a gut feel – and I'm not alone in this – and we come to that moment before we decide, where we feel like we do when we jump out of a plane or off a bungy platform – 'well, here goes!' Particularly when faced with a large, potentially life changing decision, it comes down to a moment when you follow what your being is telling you and you step forward on faith and intuition. Hopefully you are right, but you really don't know for sure.

Consider, then, if you are stressed out or in a really bad mental state where your brain is virtually scrambled, how can you step forward into a new future in that state? That is the place where bad decisions and poor outcomes are born. Conversely, if you are in a calm state and can assess all sides with due consideration, wouldn't that be a better place to decide from?

If I reflect on my own journey and back to just before I went back to Nepal and discovered yoga, if I had made a major decision at that time (if I had actually been able to) there is no doubt that it would not have ended well. After my time in Nepal, the yoga and the personal coaching which all enabled me to slow down, to listen to others, to connect with myself and what I needed, I was in a far better place to make those major decisions regarding my business and personal life.

If we look at yoga as the tool to use to help us into a better mental, emotional and spiritual space, then it is a great process to use to help us achieve better outcomes. In yoga we become quiet. We learn to listen to ourselves and connect with our inner being. We learn about ourselves and our needs and tendencies and we position ourselves better to move forward with calmness and certainty.

To be clear, yoga isn't the only way of achieving this, but this is a book designed to encourage you dudes into trying yoga, so I'm not going to miss an opportunity, am I?

My life has been full of some really major life decisions since I turned 50 and yoga has been a major contributing factor to my being able to handle them with a clear mind.

Body awareness

Guys, can you honestly say that you are very connected with and aware of your own body? Do you check in on your mental and physical state on a regular basis?

If you're anything like me, then the answer to that is most likely a resounding 'no'. There are plenty of reasons for that, but mostly it comes down to the social expectation 'toughen up and keep going' paradigm that we men often live with.

We ignore warning signs like constant muscular niggles or aches. We don't go to the doctor as often as we should. We don't take stock of our mental health, ignoring when we're constantly stressed or on edge, or not sleeping. In essence, most of us guys just operate as meat bodies moving through the universe doing our stuff, without too much thought or concern or analysis of ourselves. It's a crude analogy but I think it's pretty accurate. We are busy *doing* rather than *being*.

This general ignorance that we guys have of ourselves just sets us up for breakdowns, mentally and physically. Muscles tear, hips and knees need replacing, the doctor says it's too late for treatment, we crumble mentally, we resort to the bottle (or worse) to help us cope. We men are **pre**programmed to ignore ourselves.

But just imagine that there is a mechanism to **re**programme ourselves; a way to get us back into connection with our physical and mental selves, and improve **all** aspects of our lives as a result? Yoga is the mechanism for doing exactly that.

How can a simple activity like yoga, sitting on a rubber mat making weird shapes with our bodies, have such a profound effect on people? It's pretty simple. It's about becoming still It's about becoming quiet enough so that we can hear ourselves. What I mean by hearing ourselves is that through the act of yoga, we quieten all the internal chatter and noise, and suddenly we can hear and feel our bodies, minds, and spirits.

One of the absolute foundations of yoga, as I mentioned earlier, is the breath. By bringing our attention to our breath, we take our attention off everything else and we become able to tune in and connect to ourselves. With the additional focus and concentration on our postures, we also connect totally to our bodies. How we feel. What feels good. What feels bad. By practising yoga day after day in this quiet, connected state, we become more aware of our strengths and weaknesses. We become more aware of our bodies, where we move easily and what we struggle with.

We become better tuned into our tendencies as well. For example, you might spend the whole time in some poses just praying desperately for them to end. Once you realise this is happening, you can get curious – for maybe the first time in your life – as to why this is happening. What is it that you're struggling with? Is your body telling you that something is painful, or that it's just challeng- ing? Is your mind causing the trouble, tossing up old ideas about success and failure? How can you adjust yourself, mentally or physically, so that this changes? Get curious about the answers your body and your mind are trying to give you.

Without the quietening process, you never get closer

to learning about yourself; you just keep trucking on. A big meat body traversing through the universe in ignorance … until the breakdown. Wouldn't you rather work out how to avoid this? Wouldn't your life be better, richer, healthier and with less turmoil if you could self-manage better?

*The simple answer is to **sit down and be quiet**.*

Body discipline

How many of us guys (despite what we might say or think) are really disciplined when it comes to our bodies? Disciplined in how we exercise, what we eat, and what we feel?

Despite most of us having been involved in some sport or wellness regime at some time in our lives, I really don't think many of us have ever been or learned to be disciplined. We might go to the gym a couple of times a week, jump on the bike, or have a round of golf once in a while, but are we really engaged in our pastimes and choices?

From my perspective, I propose that the answer is 'not really', and I reckon it's because most of us guys are highly task- and goal-oriented. This matches up with the societal paradigms that we live our lives *trying* to achieve. As such, we are great if we have a big goal to work towards. For me, I know I'm pretty disciplined if I have a task set out to achieve or a goal to reach. If I know I'm heading to Nepal in six months, for example, then I'm going to consistently work at getting myself fit. I'm dedicated to that goal. It's similar in business. If I have a goal set towards achieving budgets, making things happen, getting to a new place, or whatever it is, I'm going to bust a gut to get there.

Where I'm not good is if I don't have a clear goal or if I lose sight of it. When that happens, I can very easily skip a walk or a gym session, then I can easily submit to the lure of watching a game, sitting on my arse on the couch and having a beer instead of working out.

The need to achieve a goal is really strong in us guys, and if we don't have a clear goal in mind, it can be very hard to be disciplined. Imagine if we could change things a little bit, and make it our goal to feel happy each day; to make it our intended, clear objective each day to do something that makes us feel good and is good for us?

If we look at martial arts, they are activities built on perfecting a very small action or movement before being able to move on to the next. They are really about conquering yourself and being very focused and disciplined in the pursuit of small achievements. They are broken down into bite-size pieces that you can work on incrementally and there are achievements on the way, like the belt system in karate or judo. Imagine, however, if it wasn't broken down into stages and students were expected to attain their black belt right from the start. Now, some will get there and they would be the rare few with the internal fortitude, drive and desire to do so. Most won't and they will quit as it seems unattainable.

Yoga is very much the same. Males will often look at yoga, they will see a flexible female turning herself into a pretzel and they will dismiss it as unattainable. 'I'm not flexible enough to do yoga,' is the classic excuse for a man to not even give it a try. In truth, yoga is absolutely no different to martial arts. By changing your perspective to focus on the small achievements that you make in yoga, and being disciplined enough to work toward those achievements, you will be a happier person in so many aspects of your life. The dedication to learning to understand your body better – and this comes partly by becoming very quiet and present in a yoga class – you can learn your strengths and weaknesses, and you can be gentler with yourselves and your expectations. You learn what you can and can't do and your instructor should always encourage you to work at you own level.

In truth, yoga is a life-long pursuit in personal challenge, and there is no ultimate goal. There's no gold trophy at the end, and you're not competing with anyone else. Yoga teachers refer to this as 'yoga practise'. To me, this means that you are always practising as you will never be perfect. It requires discipline to turn up to class. It requires dedication to keep working your body in ways that it isn't used to and sometimes doesn't appreciate. It requires patience.

Our bodies are all different. Some of us carry injuries or restrictions. Some have bodies that will adapt quickly to yoga, but some of us won't. What we will all experience, however, is the ability to focus more, and we will experience changes and improvements in our bodies over time. Rome wasn't built in a day, so there is no way you will get flexible overnight! Like that supermodel on the shampoo ad says, 'It won't happen overnight, but it will happen.' And it's the body discipline that yoga teaches you that will get you there.

Inner Strength

Inner strength as the ability to keep going even when it seems impossible. The ability to keep putting one foot in front of the other, despite being exhausted and not wanting to continue. The knowing that you can keep going and still have more to give.

I'd like to suggest that today's society does not promote or grow inner strength in individuals. If we look at the school system, we celebrate mediocrity. We don't let kids lose at sports or even academically because we want everyone to feel special and included, which is all lovely and nice and gives everyone the warm fuzzy feelings … until these kids go out into the real world.

Guess what? The real world is nasty. There are failures. There are people out there wanting to take what you have or stop you from getting what you want. It's tough out there, people.

I'll say one thing for the way I was bought up in the 60s. There were no warm fuzzies. It was win or lose at sport. At school you either passed or you failed. You soon learned how to deal with harsh realities, and to be honest I think it helped to prepare us better for the world.

From my experience as an employer of younger people, and from observations of the society we live in, there is a huge lacking of resilience and inner strength in people today. There is reduced tolerance for taking the knocks that life hits us with.

I can remember several younger employees who totally went to pieces if I raised my voice or expressed my displeasure with their action or performance. To be honest, I *could* be a real arsehole at times but that's not to say I was a walking disaster zone as a boss by today's standards either. There are always times when you need to sit someone down and politely but firmly correct a behaviour or method in a process to get a better result. In my humble opinion they should have easily been able to take admonishment or criticism on the chin and move on. They couldn't!

In my simple view we, as a society, no longer lay the building blocks for inner strength and resilience. There are heaps of reasons for this, from the school system right through to the reduction in kids playing team sports. Now, that is where you can learn great life lessons, including how to win and lose, but also social skills that can only be developed in team environments. They are great for developing inner strength and resilience.

Maybe you agree with me and maybe you don't, but I think it's hard to argue that we need more strong individuals in our communities who can pave their own course, and by doing so can be available to assist those who just can't for whatever reason. That's the essence of what being a community is.

Yoga can be a great catalyst for change here (you knew I was going to say that, didn't you!), and I have experienced this first hand. Yoga was the major catalyst for positive change in my life. When things were totally going to pieces for me it was the quiet and calming moments that I received in yoga classes that allowed me to take stock, regroup and refuel. Yoga really helped me build my resilience and over time it has also really helped me to understand who I am, and I know a lot of other guys who do yoga feel the same.

A yoga saying that I absolutely love is, 'yoga helps you to understand the consequences of being yourself.' Another is, 'yoga is less about tightening your arse than it is about getting your head out of it.' I love that one especially, as it really describes the state I was in just before I started yoga. I had my head right up my arse and couldn't see daylight anywhere. I was really lost and totally losing my mind. Maybe this is a feeling you know too.

Yoga helped me to see more clearly where I was and who I was by allowing me to really slow down, quiet myself and reconnect. By becoming quieter I learned to focus on the moment and the now. Prior to that I was fully focused on the 'what might happen', which at that time was soul destroying.

I became stronger by becoming more still.

This is part of the essence of yoga.

Focus

The Cambridge Dictionary defines focus as 'the main or central point of something, especially of interest or attention'. From this book's point of view, I'm going to discuss the focus of men and how focus in yoga can bring about life improvements.

As I have discussed earlier, we men largely grow up with our focus on achievement in our studies, sports and careers. As we get older this focus on career and providing becomes stronger in line with the paradigms that we grow up believing are relevant to us. We then might add a family into the mix, which doesn't necessarily change our strong focus on career, we just have more focus on providing and being successful. We also try and focus on being fit, keeping up with our sport and pastimes. More into the mix.

So, if focus is something that is central to us as males,

and as we have all of these things vying for our attention, it probably helps to explain why a lot of us struggle. We get to 40 or 50 years old with all of these separate things pulling us in all directions and we struggle to fit it all in. From a personal perspective, I really struggled and I found that my effectiveness in all aspects of my life suffered. I ended up being 70% effective in all aspects. This in itself created frustrations and to be honest I felt like a failure a lot of the time, particularly as a father. I just didn't have the energy to put much attention into my kids.

It's interesting how what can help us become most successful – focus – can end up being our downfall.

From the yoga perspective, focus is known as *drishti*. In yoga we talk about *drishti* being a focused gaze or mind. When we are in a class, we are generally so focused on the pose, the instructions and the movement, that our mind is occupied only with what we are attempting to achieve in that present moment. There is no room for thought and you can traverse through a class without your attention being demanded by anything else.

There are a few different layers of focus in yoga.

- **The physical**
  When you are new to yoga and you are not yet used to the postures your focus is bought to the purely physical or mechanical. The *drishti* will help you to maintain your balance. It will help you to find your centre and to maintain stability in your body.

- **The mental**

  Also known as focused intention. When you are in a challenging posture you may find that you start to have the desire to come out of the posture or to disassociate yourself from the posture. You might start to look around the room, scratch yourself or fidget. All of these things can take you out of the experience you are having with your body. By maintaining your *drishti* you are learning to train your mind to stay present and in the moment. You teach yourself to stay with experiences as they are happening, even if they are challenging or unpleasant. This builds your ability to do this in all areas your life. You learn to bring your focused intention into your life. Not just on the yoga mat.

- **Meditation**

  Developing the ability to sit still and quiet with the eyes open and focusing on a single point is very powerful and translates to more control of your mind and your life. It helps us to steady the endless mental chatter that we all have.

- **Focus in life**

  Having a clear vision or *drishti* can help us get to where we want to be. It helps you to have the ability to stay calm and present in difficult situations. It helps you to become less reactive and not to lash out. It helps to have a clear vision and purpose to your life. It helps to calm you when the myriad of things that we all have going on becomes too much.

Imagine having the ability to sit, quieten yourself and to bring everything into focus. Imagine being able to work through and order things methodically when demands become overwhelming. Imagine being able to find respite and refuge for an hour from your life and when you come out, having clearer focus and calmness.

This is yoga.

Yoga helps you to let go

We hold onto so many things in life, in many ways. We hold onto ideas, ideologies, feelings, emotions, hurts, people, memories and even wishes for the future. But does holding on to these things actually serve us?

Well, if we look at emotions and our past, we all know that they can have an effect on how we act and feel. An incident in earlier life can play out in emotional reactions and even physical problems, even many years later. Any chiropractor or kinesiologist will tell you that. Our body stores emotions and feelings and at (sometimes the oddest of) times they can come back to affect us – sometimes quite severely.

So, if it causes us long term problems when we *don't* let go of something that doesn't serve us particularly well as humans and individuals, I think it's pretty easy to see that when we *do* let go of whatever it is it would result in a degree of improved wellbeing and freedom. A yoga analogy is a perfect way of explaining this.

Often, we will be placed into a pose that we are not comfortable in. The body isn't quite ready for it and the first thing that we do is we start to resist the pose. Our mind starts whirring and all we can think of is how it might hurt, how hard it is, how your body *just can't do this*. We attach ourselves to the discomfort and as a result of the attachment we amplify it, often to the point where we say enough is enough and we pull out of the pose. **The essence of this is not that the pose is the problem, it's the fact that we strongly resist it**. What would happen if we just learned to calm ourselves, calm our mind, breathe into all of the sensations and just accept that this is where we are for now and that soon it will be over and it will be ok?

We can attach ourselves to all kinds of things – what may happen, what you want to happen, what you don't want to lose, what you think you need, what you like, what you don't like. According to Buddhist philosophy, attachment is the cause of misery. It causes misery because it makes us focus on the outcome of the attachment. The desire for a new house, the desire for a partner, the desire for wealth and happiness. Buddhists argue that if we let all of the attachment go and we practise non-attachment, we will find more peace and happiness.

I find it pretty hard to argue against that, but we aren't all Buddhist monks and we all have strengths and weaknesses. However, wouldn't it be great to let go of just some of the stuff in your life that no longer serves you and does not contribute to your wellbeing? This could be anything from anger towards another person or even the seemingly impossible desire to live in a house that you can't afford.

Yoga can of course help with this – yes, even this – too!

There is a pose called Lizard pose which really challenges new practitioners, as it requires a deep stretch of the hips and hamstrings and requires arm and wrist strength. I remember each time when I entered this pose how much I disliked it (my resistance started at the mere mention of the name). I'm reasonably short and muscular, so deep and wide hip and hamstring stretches really aren't on my favourites list. Often, we would go into the pose and would be told to hold it for five minutes. *'Holy shit! FIVE minutes! I'm dying here!'* I'd think. I'd fidget, I'd stay focused on all of the things I didn't want and *I couldn't wait* until the five minutes was up. As a result, my dislike persisted and each time we would go into Lizard, I felt the same way. I didn't improve.

Then one day, the teacher says, 'Don't focus on the outcome (reaching the end of the five minutes and holding a perfect pose), just focus on the process (how the body works in that position, the lengthening of the muscles, etc). Things change.'

So, I worked on the feelings in my body, my body position and how my muscles felt, and over time, slowly my body loosened up and let me in. I knew that the pose would end at some stage and I no longer focused on that five-minute end point. I stopped resisting and things improved.

Where in your life could you apply this principal of non-attachment? What can you let go of that no longer serves you?

Yoga can be a great teacher.

What we resist persists!

13

What Our Sons and Daughters Need from Us Now

There is no doubt about it, we live in strange and challenging times – with global pandemics, worldwide political uncertainty and real challenges to our planet's climate, to name a few. Not to mention the huge influence that social media exerts over our everyday life, both negatively and positively.

Where is the safety and the refuge? The certainty that our kids can have about the world and the future? Unfortunately, there really isn't a lot of certainty anywhere.

The world is really changeable and fluid. The paths that kids have today aren't as well paved as they were when I was young; you know, work hard, get an education, get a good job. It was pretty clear when I was a kid how things would pan out over our lifetimes. These days it's up for grabs. Did you know that the average tenure in one job in Australia is 3.3 years? No more job-for-life stuff.

What direction am I heading in here? Well, as parents we need to be able to give the kids the only certainty that we have within our control and that is us. We need to be solid, dependable, predictable (if that is possible for a human). The kids need to have some safety and security in their lives. We cannot do that as parents if we ourselves are unable to find stability and happiness.

So how do we achieve this? Guys, I'm speaking to you specifically.

We need to be able, first and foremost, to be very present with our kids. We need to disconnect from whatever is going on for us in our work or career and we need to devote some time and attention just to them. They need to feel special, valued and heard. I'd just like to add that I was a terrible example of this. I was so tied up in my own unhappiness and in my business that I didn't spend anywhere enough time with my children when they were young. I can recall many times when Hanan would ask if we could go fishing in the boat. Most times I'd refuse because frankly, I didn't want to as I was far too preoccupied. Do you think I regret that now? Bloody oath, I do. I'd do anything to turn that back and spend the time with him. Now, the tables are turned. He's busy and really successful and finds it hard to squeeze in time for the old man; it reminds me of the song 'The Cats in the Cradle'. Don't get me wrong, Hanan and I have a great relationship now, but I have my regrets about how I parented. We reap what we sow.

It's funny how I saw my damned business as more important than my son and daughter. I really didn't know any better. I think a lot of us guys can get caught up in that mindset. We can also get caught up in the stress and business of life in general, particularly when we get into those pivotal 40s.

So, can we change this, and how do we change this?

The answer is a resounding yes, and the way to become more present and to get away from these behaviours is to become more self-aware and surer on what we want and how we want to be.

This takes self-reflection and time understanding what it is like to be in our own skin.

We can only do that, in my opinion, if we learn to be still and to be quiet. If we stay tied up in the noise of life, we can't hear ourselves or others.

Practises such as meditation, yoga and tai chi are great for allowing us to slow down and switch off. They are also great for bringing light to the parts of ourselves that we really are unaware of, like your tendencies, your strengths and weaknesses. We become quiet and we can hear. The silence can be deafening.

We have to become very present and, in the moment, to achieve this. We learn who we are and we learn better what we want.

By learning better who we are, we are better able to give our gifts to others, especially our children. We can help develop better people and better communities. Who would have thought that yoga could have the power to change ourselves and influence others, all for the better?

You need to have walked the walk before you can talk the talk.

Why not take a walk into the yoga class and see where it leads you?

About the Author

This adventurous sportsman, mountain biker and hiker has traversed a wide range of landscapes both geographically and emotionally. By his own description, Greg Cawley is a 'normal' bloke, born and raised in New Zealand, now living in Australia, but his journey from serious entrepreneur to dedicated Yoga warrior was not one that came with safety vests or oxygen masks.

Greg started out as an audit accountant working in large corporations in the UK and Australasia. Then he 'settled into married life', buying three construction-based manufacturing companies that he grew over 23 years. Finally, he hit a wall of near failure in business and home life that resulted in depression and some significant life changes. Sadly, this is a fairly common story for men throughout and it's the hitting the wall part that Greg addresses through his own story and recovery from the wasteland of what is often termed a mid-life-crisis.

What Greg has done a little differently is that at age 55 he ceased his business career and trained to become a Yoga teacher ... but with a difference. He is not hyper flexible – suffering from injuries and physical restrictions like most men of his age. Greg's business BrikMan Yoga is also focused on bringing yoga to men with his **men only classes**. BrikMan Yoga ... Yoga for bricks ... Cos bricks don't bend. The slogan says it all 'No Sheilas. No Lycra. Just Blokes.'

Greg Cawley is on a mission is to demystify yoga for men, based on his personal experience of the amazing benefits (both physical and mental) for men who need to learn to bend so that they don't break. He also wants to inspire men of all ages to develop an attitude of selfcare, both mentally and physically for the collective benefit of all the sons and daughters who need gentle but powerful warriors in their lives.

Works Cited

Doniger, W. (2014). *On Hinduism.* Oxford University Press.

Hodges, J. L. (2007). *The Practice of Iyengar Yoga by Mid-aged Women: An Ancient Tradition in a Modern Life.* [Doctoral dissertation, University of Newcastle]. University of Newcastle Repository. https://novaprd-lb.newcastle.edu.au/vital/access/manager/Repository/uon:673

Mallinson, J., Singleton, M. (2017). *Roots of Yoga.* Penguin.

Pinch, W. R. (2006). *Warrior Ascetics and Indian Empires.* Cambridge University Press.

Ruth, A. (2015). The Health Benefits of Nose Breathing. *Nursing in General Practice, 1,* 40-42.

Singleton, M. (2010). *Yoga Body: The Origins of Modern Posture Practice.* Oxford University Press.

White, D. G. (2012). *Yoga in Practice.* Princeton University Press.

Acknowledgements

Obviously, anyone's life and a book like this is shaped by the influence of others and I'd just like to acknowledge a few people who have been very pivotal and important in my story. There are people who have helped me and who have hindered me, but when all said and done, they have all played an important part in the make-up of this story. Thank you to you all.

Huge thanks go firstly to my ex-father-in-law, Tom. Tom showed huge faith in me when it came to making the decision as to whether or not to purchase the first business. He was unflinching in his positive affirmation that I was capable of doing a good job. His faith and support were huge and I have used this example (I hope) with my own children.

Secondly, thanks in equal measure to Graeme and Zoe. Without Graeme's intuition that I was in a really bad space and his insistence that I go to Nepal, my story would have been very different. Without Zoe's kindness and generosity and the ability to really smack me in the mouth with the truth when I needed it, once again I would not be where I now am.

To my great friend Tracey who, without the many coffee chats, the truths that she faced me with, and the statement 'You have half of your life still to live, you might as well be happy,' I may well have not found that happiness.

To my brother Chris who I visited and spent weekends with regularly during my darkest times. We talked, you listened, we laughed and you kept pouring me vodkas. I don't know how much sense we made but those sessions really helped me to get through. Love ya, bro!

To my two kids, Hanan and Livia. You have no idea how grateful I am that you have followed me across the ditch to Australia. It is so good that you are close and I'm very proud of you both, although, Hanan, you need to start yoga!

To the pioneer men who show up in my classes each week. They have trusted me to take them on this journey into the largely unknown and I'm very grateful and in awe of each of you. It takes guts to try something new. Kudos to you men. Thank you, thank you, thank you.

Last and most importantly, Michelle.

Michelle saw what no one else could and she helped and nurtured me on my transition from a businessman to a yoga teacher. She helped me believe in myself and her way of constantly 'trimming' me into shape has made me a better person and hopefully a better teacher.

I'm so grateful for your gentle persistence, your perseverance and patience and your love.

Case Studies

CD is a semi-retired farmer in his 60s who came to yoga because someone else he knew had also started, and he thought it might complement what he was already doing at the gym.

> CD: 'I really liked the first session because it was so low key, and not formal the way I imagined women's classes are. So, I felt good from the start.'

Having had a small issue with sciatica, he noticed after only a few sessions of yoga that it just wasn't there anymore. Neither was the ongoing nagging problem of a sore back when standing for any long periods of time. Being able to turn around in his seat was noticeably easier, especially when flying in planes – a regular thing for him in his work. As he continued to notice the little things like increased flexibility and the lack of those niggly issues, CD has determined that yoga has been hugely beneficial to his overall physical and mental health. Yoga classes have even taken precedence over his gym attendance if he has felt any additional physical issues arise such as a sore knee.

CD had gone to a couple of women's yoga classes and did not enjoy those, feeling they were far more formal than he felt comfortable in, and he felt that the poses were impossible to do with his current ability. He said it was particularly hard watching a limber young female instructor who clearly had advanced flexibility on her side, and this only served to make him feel older and clumsier in that environment with so many women. It simply didn't feel achievable.

CD's friend suggested trying yoga for blokes only and from the start it was enjoyable, and the other guys in the class seemed 'more like me' with various injuries and restrictions he could easily relate to.

CD: I love most that I am more flexible so that sitting, standing, and doing general activities that in some instances I was starting to slow down on are easier. Simply stretching and learning the routine that feels better each and every time is great. If you talk to a woman about yoga, they get all enthusiastic but don't seem to get that we have different ways of wanting to push ourselves physically. For any guy thinking about yoga, they think they have to be a certain size or have certain physical abilities, but really, this is for all kinds of men. Once you feel the benefits it's hard to turn back from it. And you quickly stop thinking about what every other guy in the class is doing or thinking because you're only really challenging yourself. It's your own yoga.

BT is a fit, 45-year-old tradie who spent time in the Amazon jungle, where he was first introduced to meditation. He thought, when the idea first came up, to just see what happened and was quickly drawn into the idea of it, despite thinking of himself as primarily resistant to such things.

BT: You soon find yourself listening to more ideas from a range of people. Some say that walking in bare feet is a good way to ground yourself and so it's good for your mind and soul. I think that's true, because you become open to seeing and hearing things differently and sometimes that's a really good thing.

Nowadays, BT uses the meditations in yoga class to help keep him centred and actively mindful of his own states. Feeling pissed off is something he notices more, rather than just getting into that state of being. Awareness of his tendencies to anxiety or aggravation has also helped him to gravitate more towards acting on his feelings of kindness towards others.

BT: *I think it's more about allowing and just letting things wash over you more than just reacting to everything. I just feel like I'm a better person for having this time out to be consistent with my body care and mindfulness.*

MT is a fit, 40-year-old self-employed carpenter who came to yoga mainly in order to become more flexible. Years of heavy lifting had started to tell on his back, and after a six-week adjustment program followed by ongoing treatments that ultimately added to his pain, he started to lose faith in medical options over six months of treatment. He had previously invested in a home gym but hardly ever used it. He happened to see some of my posts on Facebook about yoga and something clicked one day, so he signed up for an introductory set of classes.

MT: I've been told from the doctor that it would probably need surgery. Although surgery can fix it, it could still take 12 months to recover from which is really not practical with the hands-on job that I do. I also went to a physio but was getting nowhere and I felt I was getting bad advice.

Greg encouraged me to work within my own boundaries and slowly it has improved and I'm confident physically in all poses now, despite having started a bit rough with some of them. Also, with the trust I was able to put in him and his teaching, I discovered I had increased confidence in myself because I can control how far I want to push it. I'm in charge of my own yoga practise.

MT has noticed a huge change in his overall flexibility; some things have developed more slowly than others, and he's noticed that he's getting better about just breathing and staying present. Arguments at home have taken a different turn as he feels more confident about just not engaging in drama and emotional challenges that come up with family members.

MT: I have become more aware of my reactions. I would never before have been able to just breathe and become present and not escalate a problem – mentally I'm much better at blocking out all the other thoughts about what someone else might think about me or what I think about them. I'm in my own space, my own bubble. That doesn't mean I ignore things, but I'm more in control of how I deal with things.

MT also believes he physically looks better, has more muscle tone, and is mentally stronger too. And as he's been overheard to say that, living with three women (wife and daughters), his yoga hour and time with other blokes is a highlight of his week. Hooked on the many benefits, he's now trying to get his dad to start yoga too.

BC is a 42-year-old stay-at-home dad who was battling severe depression, anxiety and schizophrenia when he started yoga. His wife had suggested he needed to do something, sensing he was reaching a tipping point and he was ready to 'try anything'.

BC is 60 kilos lighter, and feels he's coping better, and has even been able to reduce his medication, which he credits to his yoga 'mental nap time'. He says he's learned to zone out and focus better on what he *can* control, through the combination of yoga and working with a new psychiatrist.

> *BC: I'm on the right path now. Not perfect but on the right path. That is attributed in part to going to yoga once or twice a week. It gets me that mental nap time.*
>
> *I still take pharmaceutical medication but not as much as before. I haven't turned to drugs or alcohol. I have been strong enough not to do that. I'm also involved now with a new psychiatrist. But at least I made a start in this new direction and that comes down to the tipping point of starting to do yoga.*
>
> *The mental side of it has been huge for me. Just to be open to the achievements that I make and to focus on just a day-to-day basis. Being able to better to deal with situations. Just to focus on breathing and being more grounded and learning how to cope with things.*

BC also feels that his previous anger issues are radically improved due to being able to think more clearly, let go of negative and pent-up energy, and he feels looser and more flexible.

BC: Being present and quiet and aware of your surroundings. But I think being in touch with your breathing and to control your breathing is really beneficial. It's hard to describe. It's just created an overall better feeling of wellbeing. You just feel better. I walk into a class feeling good and when I walk out, I feel amazing.

All our case study fellas have said these same things:

They would likely not have walked into a female yoga class, but love the men's only options because they get 'yoga time out' and there are no distractions for that time. Some dislike some of the poses, but all agree that it's the same doing any kind of exercise – there's always going to be something that's less favourite and that you quickly get used to the poses and can measure your progress against yourself doing them.

Some commented that in many ways everyone has some kind of mental health or crisis point in life at some time or other. How you deal with it is what makes the difference in how you survive those times. Yoga has been credited with helping that process through teaching how to be calm, centred, and present. Breathing and a better sense of being in control is only one of the benefits – all have also seen improvements in their physical wellbeing too.

And all the fellas I talk to about yoga say this: Once you've tried it, you're going to be surprised how much you love it. And you surely will love it a lot!

Disclaimer: While many of my clients have found yoga helpful, I do not suggest yoga as an alternative to mental health treatments. Please seek medical advice if you feel you need help with any medical or mental health matters.

If you'd like to join me on a yoga mat sometime, now is always a good time for Yoga – and we can do this in person or from anywhere in the world thanks to the modern option of zoom and online classes

Check out my website
www.gregcawleyyoga.com.au

For in studio classes and to book your spot
www.gregcawleyyoga.com.au/classes

Join me for online Zoom classes at (these classes are growing and evolving as we sort out the technology)
www.gregcawleyyoga.com.au/zoom

Enrol in my online 4 module Introduction to Yoga Course (Ideal for those of you new to yoga and wanting to dip your toe in the water)
www.gregcawleyyoga.com.au/intro

Follow Brikman Yoga on facebook
www.facebook.com/brikmanyoga

Follow Brikman Yoga on Instagram #brikmanyoga

Contact me via my website for enquiries related to one-on-one training, customised workshops, or to speak at your event.

And finally guys, whatever you do, take this momentum and get yourself to a yoga class no matter where you are.

Your mind and body will love you for it!

Greg